Signs of Life

This is an IndieMosh book

brought to you by MoshPit Publishing
an imprint of Mosher's Business Support Pty Ltd

PO Box 4363
Penrith NSW 2750

indiemosh.com.au

NATIONAL LIBRARY OF AUSTRALIA

A catalogue record for this work is available from the National Library of Australia

nla.gov.au/collections

Title:	Signs of Life
Subtitle:	An anthology
Edited by:	Sasson, Sarah (1979–)
ISBNs:	978-1-922542-86-1 (paperback) 978-1-922542-55-7 (ebook – epub) 978-1-922542-56-4 (ebook – mobi)
Subjects:	BIOGRAPHY & AUTOBIOGRAPHY: Medical (incl. Patients); MEDICAL: Caregiving; MEDICAL: Physician & Patient; FAMILY & RELATIONSHIPS: Death, Grief, Bereavement; MEDICAL: Mental Health

Cover image copyright © 2018 Melanie van Kessel at melanievankessel.com/

Cover layout by Ally Mosher at allymosher.com

Signs of Life

— an anthology

Edited by

Sarah Sasson

Foreword

How do experiences of sickness or incapacitation change our bodies, who we are, and how we see the world? And how do they affect the people around us?

In 2018 I'd relocated to Oxford, UK, with my husband and young children to take up a research position. In between starting a new job, settling the kids into day-care and setting up the house, these were the ideas I was ruminating on. At the time they seemed like somewhat niche concerns; I knew I was drawn to them as someone who'd studied biological/medical science and literature, but would other people be interested in reading an anthology themed on first- and second-hand experiences of illness and care giving? I wasn't sure.

One of the first steps I took was to contact illustrator Melanie van Kessel. I'd found some of her beautiful hand-drawn works online and I emailed her to ask if she would be interested in working on the project. In her response Melanie let me know that she had only recently returned to her art after a long medical recovery period. *How fitting* I thought, *that the illustrator has such a recent and personal connection to the theme.*

She wasn't the only one. During the six-month call-out period I received nearly 200 submissions including from: Australia, Canada, the USA, the UK, Ireland, India, Switzerland, Taiwan, Trinidad and Tobago, Nigeria, Chile, Pakistan and Indonesia. Within them a myriad of situations and conditions were explored, each told from a distinct vantage point. What struck me was how many of the works dealt with neurological, psychological and psychiatric issues: anxiety, delusions, dementia, depression, bipolar disorder, post-traumatic stress disorder, Parkinson's disease, schizophrenia, migraines, stroke and vertigo among them. Was this simply reflective of the high prevalence of these diseases in the community? Perhaps. For the person with the condition, these are illnesses that can change the perception of the world as they move through it; those in care giving roles can face a compounded loss: not only of their patient's or loved one's wellbeing but even sometimes seeming to lose parts of who they were, either transiently, or not. As my inbox filled up it was apparent: these were vital stories that demanded to be told.

In their submission letters writers were asked to nominate which point of view they were writing from: patient, care giver (professional or otherwise) or kin. It was an oversight on my behalf, one that I realised when many of the submissions returned classified as "carer/kin". What a common pattern it is to slip into a care giving role for our children, parents and partners. A strange dance we subconsciously move through as we disassemble what relationship we had and build it into something else. The related grief is often intense and invisible.

From an initial longlist of outstanding entries, the final selection was made. I notified the authors in January 2020 from my mother's apartment back in Sydney where we stayed briefly after our return. Our two-year stint in the UK had come to an end. It was the start of a new year and I was looking forward to going to the beach, catching up with friends and family and starting new projects. I had no sense of what was just around the corner.

In February of 2020, I watched with vague interest the first reports of a novel virus originating from Wuhan, China, and wondered if the course would be similar to that of the original SARS virus, or MERS, neither of which had a high incidence in Australia. By early March my husband and I sat on the couch horrified at footage of Italian hospitals being overwhelmed. Wards and corridors were clogged with gurneys, elderly patients struggled to breathe, some sat up with large bubble-like helmets covering their heads. 'It's coming for us,' my husband, an intensive care specialist, said with his eyes locked on the screen. A few weeks later he intubated the first COVID-19 patient in his unit. As an immunologist who spent the majority of my time in diagnostic pathology, I was not one of the most exposed clinicians at the hospital where I worked. My name was added to a list of physicians that would be called on if the frontline became 'depleted'.

The contributing authors and I moved through the editing

process at a time when much of the globe was in lockdown. The way we wrote to each other changed. We did not open emails with an assumption that things would be found well, but instead asked *how are things where you are*? Instead of *best wishes* to sign off we wrote *take care*. Or *keep safe*.

As we go to press much of the world remains in various states of tragedy, chaos, disarray and lockdown. But there is also hope; the fast-turning wheels of science and industry have provided us with three approved COVID-19 vaccines in the Western world and with more on the horizon globally. I read with interest about the first vaccine recipient in England, a 90-year-old woman from Coventry. When I saw the image of her sleeved rolled over shoulder, the pale flash of her upper arm as the jab went in, I thought of the many challenges and disappointments she must have faced and overcome and for a moment wondered with amazement that a zoonotic bat virus might have been added to the ledger.

In this collection you will spend time with people living with chronic pain, HIV infection, undergoing spinal surgery and being treated for cancer. There are compelling accounts of living with Tourette's' Syndrome, bipolar disorder and other mental health challenges.

The depicted carers are often caught in double binds: between providing much-needed help but against aggressive intractable disease course, while navigating the intricacies of healthcare systems, or while in foreign countries. Doctors and other health professionals in these pages provide care while being overcome with the emotional toll of the job, through facing their own private challenges, or despite they themselves being incapacitated.

While I anticipated publishing stories that dealt with the challenge and hardship of being unwell, or caring for those afflicted, *Signs of Life* was never intended to be a book on death and dying. This is an anthology about life and how we live it, at the gritty interface between our most basic needs and the relationships that define us.

Three years since first asking questions about illness and caregiving, and those ideas I initially thought of as fringe have consumed all of us for the past year. What has editing this anthology shown me? More than anything, that the shock of illness or incapacitation brings with it great clarification. Suddenly all the busy details of everyday retreat and we see with great clarity what it is we need to survive. Sustenance. Rest. Love. Possibilities. There is no easy or right way to be a carer, and especially a kin/carer. These are roles that are difficult at a macro level as they involve inversions of relationships, grieving the loss of what was, putting to the side one's prior ambitions or purpose to tend to another's needs; but also frustrating at the more micro level, like trying to manoeuvre a wheelchair out from a small room, or care for someone who is lashing out. How do you communicate to the world who your child with autism is and how to understand their difference? How do we adequately care for our parent? Doctors, nurses and other health professionals face distinct challenges in pursuing their vocation. Being a health care worker means dedicating your life to the service of others, to witnessing their suffering through illness and sometimes feeling complicit in regards to any adverse effects of their treatment. It is a job that is often physically and emotionally taxing, and one that does not always ensure psychological safety. In dedicating our working lives to tending to others, how do we ensure we care also for ourselves? And when health professionals become overwhelmed or incapacitated how do they transition to being a patient? Indeed, how well do any of us move between the roles of patient, care giver or family member?

The organisation and collation of this anthology was something that required a significant amount of time and effort, most of which occurred in the evenings and on the weekend. Despite all the energy I invested into this collection, every time I returned to it, somehow it gave me back more.

What I've come to understand is that signs of life are not the ember-like, flickering remains that follow illness, they are our determined hope-filled actions—what we reach out, against all odds and cling to, or who.

Sarah Sasson
Editor, *Signs of Life*
January 2021

A note on content

This book contains subject matter that may be triggering for some readers. This includes cancer, death, dementia, eating disorders, medical procedures, mental illness, self-harm and suicide. Additionally, details related to particular medical conditions are described. For these reasons an index is provided at the back of the book that denotes sensitive material that is covered in individual pieces.

Please also note the anthology contains pieces from Australia, the UK, USA, and Canada among other places. An editorial decision has been made to keep the different versions of English for each individual piece.

Contents

Create It Away

Katie Danis

The first time I got my leg stuck in a broken drainpipe, I was naked. As my preschool teacher dismantled the pipe to free my entrapped—and freshly nude—limb, a new crease crept from her cheek to her chin. She was twenty-five and had eight wrinkles; at the beginning of the school year, she'd had zero. (In my defense, I held direct responsibility for only seven.)

When my parents regaled Dr McGoogan with my laundry list of strange behaviors,[1] he smiled rows of perfect teeth. I caught words in their discussion: 'creative', 'neurodivergent' and 'comorbidity'—nice words with sharp t's to tap out with your tongue. As I sat on my hands and swung my legs, my eyes wandered over the upside-down scrawl on his sheet: *Diagnosis: Tourette Syndrome.*

Tourette Syndrome, also known as Tourette's or TS, is a neurological condition 'characterized by repetitive, stereotyped, involuntary movements and vocalizations called tics' (National Institute of Neurological Disorders and Stroke). The condition was named for the French neurologist Dr Georges Gilles de la Tourette, who defined it in 1885. TS involves at least one vocal tic. It is hereditary and comorbid with OCD and ADHD. (If you have all three, congratulations! You win a can of Campbell's Neuropsychological Alphabet Soup.) Approximately 200,000 Americans live with TS.

---

[1] Including, but not limited to, banging my head on the floor for hours without cause, hunching over like Quasimodo and clawing out my eyebrows, randomly shrieking as if in imitation of a stoned screech owl's mating call (and doing a bang-up job, if you ask me), raising my eyebrow, furrowing my eyebrow, blinking 'SOS' in Morse code, compulsively inhaling underwater, touching my palm to the pavement in the middle of a busy street, and furiously flapping my arms like a forty-pound brunette penguin poised to storm a fishery. You know, normal kid stuff.

I would learn all of this later.

For years, I knew Tourette's as a personal intracranial beast. Mostly I thought of it as my built-in brain gremlin, but it could be a shapeshifter. Its voice commanded me to bang my head and clear my throat and twist my eyebrows until the hairs pirouetted like helicopter seeds. Yet the voice told me to do not-so-suffocating things, too. To spin in the rain until the world smeared like watercolors. To scale beech trees despite my fear of heights. To investigate a shattered drainpipe on the playground. (For the record, the school gave me an award for exposing the drain as a health hazard. However, the accolade's name—the Nudie Beauty Award—somewhat undermined its resumé potential.[2]) I breathed adventure, ticking and ticcing towards the next discovery like a neurotic Indiana Jones. No matter how many times I lost my path, the chatter of compulsions and curiosities followed me through the maze: a constant, if unsolicited, companion in exploration.

The DSM-5 classifies Tourette's as a tic 'disorder', a problem that requires treatment. Something broken. Something not-quite-right. Something you can pinch and tuck and drown in Xanax and proclaim, 'All better.' Dr McGoogan and my parents carefully floated words towards each other like day-old helium balloons, stiffly volleying them as they trembled in the air. I glanced back at the sheet, turning the diagnosis over in my mouth. *Tourette*. It tasted French, and I liked that. I also liked that it contained the word 'tour', because a tour promised an adventure: an old-smelling art gallery, a rain-scented path through a tangle of beech trees, or, best of all, a library with a twisty staircase like the one in *Beauty and the Beast.* I lived for the labyrinth: sometimes I was Theseus; sometimes I was Daedalus; always I was David Bowie, magic-dancing through the shelves.

However, not all magic twirls through tangled bookshelves and sings in the rain and sparkles like fairy dust and releases chart-topping

---

[2] I tried slipping the award onto my college application before the school counselor shut me down. Honestly, I'm more proud of this achievement than any other, including the time I ate nine Saltine crackers in one minute without water. That's three quarters of a world record.

reggae fusion singles.[3] The voice in my head is my curse. I felt like Princess Aurora in *Sleeping Beauty*: bewitched at birth to prick my finger on a spindle (again and again and again and again). But *this* curse lurked in my DNA, incurable by kiss (true love's or another kind) or prescription. I wondered if a demon lived inside me, and the Catholic officiaries in my community did not help to ease this suspicion, instead reprimanding me for asking too many questions in Sunday school ('If Noah's ark landed in ancient Mesopotamia after Pangea fractured, then how did wallabies get to Australia?'[4]) and for repeatedly clearing my throat during Communion. I became a disciple of loneliness. I spent so much time practicing guilt that relief tasted like giving up.

There's a saying that goes something like, *You are never so alone as in a crowd.* Tourette's has a way of making you feel alone, like you're onstage squinting through the spotlights at an audience who won't look you in the eye. When I tic in church, I am alone. When I tic in school, I am alone. When I tic at the supermarket or the committee meeting or the hardware store, in the library or the parking lot or the elevator, at the soccer game or the Christmas party or Carnegie Hall, I am alone. Then I feel a different kind of lost, the kind that makes you hug your knees as the path lies before you, all bright and alive, and just stare, stare, stare.

The kind of lost where you don't want to be found.

So I discovered ways to lose myself. When I funneled all of my focus into an activity, the tics lessened. The voice in my head did not go entirely mum, but it quieted. Stilled. Listened. When I sang, the gremlin nodded its head to the beat. When I wrote, my fingers danced and twitched about the keyboard like a glitching Franz Liszt.[5] When

---

3 Fun fact: the band Magic! recently joined Samantha Bee, Kiefer Sutherland and Alex Trebek on my running list 'Canadian Celebrities Whose Nationality I Was Surprised to Discover Because of My American Egocentrism'.

4 The answer, of course, is that wallabies made a pact with Satan to join the pantheon of demons now running free in the Australian Outback. The Wallapocalypse is coming. Don't deny it, for deep down you always knew it to be true.

5 Note to self: 'Glitching Franz Liszt' isn't a bad band name.

I ran, my legs windmilled in a familiar ticcing rhythm, the gremlin heaving and straining until, eventually, it fell into pace. In those breezy moments, I was free.

Of course, exercising my creativity will not exorcise the voice in my head. I could sprint from Greensboro to Galilee[6] and Ol' Faithful Azazel[7] would be waiting for me at the finish line. I will never outrun my demons. All I can do is enter the labyrinth again and again, and Bowie knows it isn't a day outing. However, I've realized the mutations that condemn me to glitch like a virus-infected Lenovo ThinkPad also instill in me insatiable curiosity and an obsessive drive to improve the world. (Not to mention a proclivity for punning that may incite my brother to strangle me one day. I can't help but put some antics in semantics.[8]) Like Harry Potter's psychic connection with Voldemort, my curse is also my greatest blessing—except, unlike Harry, I can't innately speak to snakes; I had to take a class.[9]

Here's the thing: everyone's fighting something. That's one of two things I know for sure. (The other is that oatmeal raisin cookies were created by the Communist Party of the Soviet Union during the Cold War to lower American morale. They look like chocolate chip cookies and taste like trust issues, and that's a fact.) But in my extremely short time as a moderately successful human, if we measure success by the amount of peanut butter a person can consume in one sitting,[10] I find that the worst of human experience can bring out the best of human ingenuity. Not in the case of the oatmeal raisin cookie, but sometimes. I accept that the voice in my head is here to stay and, more importantly, that I don't want it to leave. I'm rather attached to

---

6 Note to self: 'Greensboro to Galilee' is a better band name.

7 Note to self: 'Ol' Faithful Azazel' is the best band name.

8 After reading that line, my dear brother dropped the pages of this essay on the floor and walked away.

9 Jest notwithstanding, four-year-old Katie really did want to become a snake charmer—specifically in Cairo for its cool mummies and cheap real estate.

10 I'm up to a respectable 1.4 midsize jars, which roughly translates to 25 ounces. Please hold your applause.

it. Besides, it gets lonely in the labyrinth, so it's nice to have the Minotaur—Minotourette?—for company.

When I say that getting lost is my greatest gift, I receive a dismissive waving of hands. 'Nice try, Katie. Your inability to locate your living room without Google Maps[11] is not a superpower.'

But the subtle art of losing yourself is just that—an art, the product of excess creative energy that can be channeled through piano-playing, marathon-running, poetry-writing, opera-singing, and the occasional drainpipe misadventure. *Disorder* implies *wrong*, but there is no right way to be. Heredity gave me a reservoir of nervous energy, and rather than dulling it with Dexedrine, I run faster, write longer, sing higher, am kinder. I create it away. The alleles that urge me to touchthefloortouchthefloortouchthefloor also afford me laser-like focus, allowing me to lose myself in letters, people, paintings. I get lost to find myself and to live with the self I find. The tics and twitches are me like my matrimonial devotion to Justin's Chocolate Hazelnut Butter is me, or my passion for making academic rap videos is me, or my use of the vocative comma in email greetings is me, or my desire to befriend both Oscar Wilde and Ernest Hemingway so I can make jokes about 'the importance of being Ernest'[12] is me. I do not succeed despite my condition; I succeed[13] because of it, and to mute it is to blunt my creativity, my curiosity, the core of my identity.

When Dr McGoogan propelled a stale red balloon across his desk with an *Rx* scribbled behind a boldfaced question mark, my mom stood up. She plucked the question out of the air and squeezed. It popped with a flat crack, and she flicked it onto the floor. As she strode towards the door, tugging my dad along, she paused. Turned. Smiled. 'Let's go, Katie,' she said. And for once in my life, I obeyed.

---

[11] This joke is uncomfortably close to the truth. It's hard to overstate the extent of my navigational incapacity.

[12] This zinger has been stewing in my head for two years and change. Only problem is, there are by my calculations approximately zero situations that would warrant its public appearance. Darn.

[13] Again, assuming success is positively correlated with nut butter consumption. Which it obviously is.

The first time I got stuck in a broken drainpipe was not the last. I walk into the labyrinth again and again, a restless adventurer getting lost, trying and testing and ticcing while knowing that I'll never get out, that I don't want to, that all I can do is stand at the crossroads of *was* and *will* and explore the maze in between. If I am wrong, at least I am myself. That's the only life I want to live.

Now, if you'll excuse me, I need to find my way down from this tree.

The Man from Saint Jude's

Janey Runci

The bare limbs of the liquidambar in her back garden were only just visible in the mist, like ghostly arms hovering. She stood at the window, on that morning her son was to go to Saint Jude's, her dressing-gown wrapped tight around her and a cup of hot tea in her hands. Even with the heater on she couldn't get warm.

Finally she knocked on her son's bedroom door. When there was no answer she waited a while and knocked again, and when he still didn't answer she pushed the door open. The blind was down, but she could see he was lying just as he had a few hours before when she'd last tended to him, his dark head on the pillow, the length of his body under the blanket. He was a tall man; this was only really noticeable when he was lying down rather than in his wheelchair. His eyes were open, staring up at the ceiling.

'Hi,' she said.

'Get out,' he said.

'Do you want me to turn you?'

'I said, get out.'

~

An hour later, two burly men arrived with the patient transport van. They hoisted her son from his bed into his chair. He resisted all the way, as much as he was able, while she stood there babbling. 'It's only for two weeks. We both need a rest. I'm sorry. I'm sorry.'

The men worked calmly and efficiently as though there was nothing unusual happening. They slipped the hoist straps from under her son's body and adjusted him in his wheelchair. Perhaps they knew that the team who had been caring for her son while she was at work had recently refused to continue in this role. Perhaps they knew that he had pinned one carer up against the wall in his electric chair, but maybe they didn't. Or maybe it didn't matter to them.

One of the men patted her arm and said, 'You could get his bag, love.'

When they got to the front door her son looked at her directly for the first time that morning and said, 'Don't bother to come. I hate you, and I'm going to take legal action against you.'

'Now, now, son,' one of the men said.

'I'm sorry,' she said again. 'I'm sorry.'

~

The house was deathly quiet after the patient transport van drew away. She walked from one room into another and back again, and finally she sat in the old armchair and stared out the window. The mist was clearing, weak sun breaking through.

She could hear the clock ticking. Nine-thirty. The van would be at Saint Jude's. She got up. She took hold of a dining chair and lifted it, held it there, poised, for what? To throw it through the large picture window? To hear and see the splintering glass, the chair flying on, the house made open to the garden, to the sky, and her standing there, howling.

She stood like that for a minute or more, then she lowered the chair—not to the floor, but to the top of the table, setting it there among what was left of breakfast. She took hold of another chair and put it there too, and the four or five remaining chairs around the table, moving quicker and quicker with each chair. She began to load furniture of all kinds on top of other furniture: small tables on armchairs, cushions on top of that. She gathered up the piles of books and magazines and newspapers from the floor. She was clearing the floor. She was going to have a big clean.

She stood there, surveying it all, when the front doorbell rang. It was probably a staff member from one of the agencies who didn't know that her son had this very morning gone to Saint Jude's. It was unlikely to be any of her friends; they had learnt to phone before they came over.

She stared out the back window again. Time passed, and she began to imagine that the visitor had gone, but the bell rang again, long and slow, as if the visitor was holding their hand on the button. Perhaps it was the postman. She went slowly up the passage, trying to identify the head she could see through the pane of frosted glass in the top part of the door: a head belonging to an older man who was tall, but that was as much as she could tell.

As she hesitated behind the door, the bell rang again and she jumped. He bent forward and pressed his face to the glass. When she opened the door, he stood there holding a large white envelope. He stared at her, steadily.

'What are you doing here?' she said.

'I wanted to see you, to ask you to do something for me.'

It was like being in a film, and she was playing a lead role, but she couldn't remember what it was.

He held the envelope towards her. 'I will pay you the full rate.'

If it was a film the envelope would be full of banknotes, but she knew this one wasn't. It was the kind of envelope used to hold a manuscript, and the visitor was the elderly Jewish man from her writing class.

'You should have made an appointment at the college,' she said. 'You shouldn't have come to my house. How do you know where I live?'

He lifted his hands as if to say that was another story, while one hand kept holding the large envelope towards her.

'You have to go away,' she said.

'It won't take long.' He was leaning closer, the way he did when he was telling stories in class.

He was the student who stood out in her class that year: a commanding storyteller, at least orally. He came to class dressed formally as he was now, in a jacket and a tie and old-fashioned leather shoes, freshly polished. He always stood to deliver even the shortest narrative. He had a way of surveying the class before he spoke. He knew when to pause and when to wait. Sometimes when he rose to speak, she wanted to call out, *Listen to this man! This man knows what a story is. This man knows how to tell it!*

And now, on this day her son was taken to Saint Jude's, he stood at her front door with an envelope in his hand.

'This is a very bad day in my life,' she said.

'It won't take long, if you let me come in.'

And then somehow he stepped forward and she stepped back and he came into her house. They walked down the passage to the room where all the furniture was in crazy piles, all of them seeming about to slip down.

He lifted one of the chairs from the dining table and then another. 'We'll sit,' he said.

~

What he wanted was for her to take the manuscript of the story of his life and fix it. Those were the words he used: 'You can fix it. You know how.'

It was a lengthy manuscript; she could see that from the thickness of the envelope.

'I can't,' she said.

'I will pay you more than the rate. You could use the money?'

They sat facing each other on their dining chairs. He pulled out his wallet. There were several hundred-dollar notes in it. She knew that he and his wife were living in a small flat and on a meagre stipend, both provided by a Jewish benevolent society.

'You know my heart is bad?' he said.

She knew he'd been hospitalised for a week or more earlier in the year. She nodded.

'So it is urgent that you do this,' he said. He began to remove the manuscript from the envelope.

'This is maybe the worst day of my life,' she said.

He kept easing the manuscript out.

'My son has been taken away,' she said. 'I arranged for him to be taken away. To a place called Saint Jude's.'

'Your son in the wheelchair?' the man said, as though she had sons to spare. 'They will care for him there.'

'Saint Jude's,' she said again. 'Saint Jude is the patron saint of the despairing. Did you know that?'

He shook his head. 'Is there another place he could go?'

'Not for his needs.'

'I see.' He finished pulling the manuscript out and laid the cover page in front of her.

She stared down at it. The words made no sense. She stared and stared and then she shook her head. 'I can't!' She went to stand up, but her legs felt too weak. 'This place—Saint Jude's—a man who was staying there, he drove his own wheelchair over the escalator.' She paused, her breath coming fast. 'At Chadstone.'

'Chadstone?' For the first time in his visit, he seemed to pause. His hands went loose. The manuscript lay on the table. 'Should we have a cup of tea?'

'I can't do it,' she said.

'The tea or the manuscript?'

'Anything.'

'I see.' And he did seem to see for the first time: the heaped-up furniture, the used breakfast dishes, the laundry piled at her son's bedroom door. 'I will make the tea.' He stood up. 'And you will tell me about this man from Saint Jude's.'

~

She took a sip from her cup then sat for a moment. 'It happened at Chadstone Shopping Centre,' she said finally, 'on a group outing from St Jude's.' She stopped, staring down at her milky tea.

'Would it help if you stood?' he said.

She felt as though her legs wouldn't hold her, but when she pushed herself up from the chair, they did. He moved his own chair back a little to listen.

'A man in the group …' she said.

He nodded, serious.

'In his wheelchair …'

'Yes.'

'This man moved away from the group towards the escalator, the steep one, the downward-travelling one.'

'I know it,' he said.

'Nobody from the group saw this. They were looking in the pet-shop window, at the new puppies and kittens. They had their backs to him.'

'Yes.'

'As he got closer to the escalator he must have bent forward in his chair.' She was bending forward herself. 'His hands moved quicker and quicker on the spinning wheels.' Her hands were mimicking the motion. 'A man from security saw what was happening, but it was too late …'

He stared at her, intently, unmoving.

'The man in his chair went flying over the top,' she said.

He closed his eyes briefly. 'That is awful,' he said as he opened them. 'To die like that, but that is what he wanted?'

'He didn't die.'

'But you said he went flying over the top.'

'That's how the story was told, that he went flying.'

'You weren't there?'

'No. Someone told me, just after I agreed to send my son to Saint Jude's. I think about it all the time, and it wouldn't have been like flying. It wouldn't.'

'No?'

'No! It'd be like tumbling and then jamming into the side, then tumbling again, and people screaming, mothers covering their children's eyes, people rushing to the foot of the escalator, and someone yelling for security and someone turning the escalator off and that tips the chair forward, almost upside down, the man hangs strapped in his chair, his head about to slam into the stairs …'

He held out his hand. 'Sit down.' His hand was large and warm as he took her cold and shaking one. He helped her to sit. 'You stay there,' he said. 'I'll find something to eat.'

~

'They think it will be like flying,' she said.

'Who do?' He handed her a plate of biscuits.

'The man from Saint Jude's. Our children. My son.'

He considered this. 'Have you ever wanted to fly?'

'Me?' She hadn't thought of this. 'I suppose so, when I was young. Like all kids I jumped off chairs and boxes, flapping my arms.'

He smiled. 'My children did that.'

His hand lay on the manuscript on the table between them. She already knew much of the story in its pages, a story of epic proportions: a small boy of nine, son of a rabbi, in a large, hungry family in a Polish village, turned out to fend for himself; years of scrounging to survive and then the horror of a concentration camp; his escape from the camp, and a long and hazardous journey to this country where he settled with his wife and children.

'But sometimes it is hard with our children,' he said.

This was the other part of his story, in one way the last chapter or rather the second-last chapter because there was also this present chapter in which he'd written the story. In the second-last chapter, living finally in what felt like a safe country with his children grown into adulthood, he went guarantor to his daughter and son-in-law's purchase of a home. They were not able to keep up the repayments, and in the end the man's own home was lost. In the acrimony that followed the daughter and son-in-law cut off contact with the man and his wife, who were now elderly and dependent on a benevolent society; they were even denied contact with their grandchildren. Now he had written his story in the hope that one day his grandchildren would read it.

'You always want to help your children, to save them from danger,' he said. 'But will it help if you get sick in the mind like you are now?'

'Pardon?'

'You can't avoid the sorrow,' he said, 'but one thing I have learnt …' He held one arm out to the side. 'If my child needs help …' He lifted the other arm and brought it down in a chopping movement on the first arm. 'I will cut off my arm for them.' He paused again, as he often did when he was telling a story in class, though this time he remained seated. He leaned towards her. 'But only …' He paused a third time. 'Only if it will help them, only then.' He stared at her. 'You understand what I am saying?'

~

After the man left the house she stood at the back window. Outside the mist had completely cleared, and the wet bare branches of the liquidambar gleamed in the sunlight like graceful limbs, and she remembered something that had happened a few years before her son's accident, before he was in a wheelchair, something she had not thought of for a long time.

When her son was about seventeen, he went missing for some months. The police were unhelpful; they pointed out that this was not uncommon for young men. She pestered them until they made it clear they'd done as much as they were going to do.

One day when she came home from work and turned into the yard, she saw something move on the front verandah. There were about six steep steps up to the verandah, and a large camellia bush grew beside the steps. A flash of colours moved away from the dark green of the camellia leaves. The colours were earthy—orange and sienna and ochre—and as she watched they unfurled and it was her son in a poncho and he called to her and then he leaped from the top step and his long black curls lifted and the poncho flew out like wings and for a moment he was caught there in the late afternoon light.

On the day her son went to Saint Jude's she stood at the window, staring out at the tree for some time, before she turned back to the room. She couldn't help but smile then, when she saw the manuscript on the table.

She gathered her bag, her car keys, and some fruit to take to her son. She set off for Saint Jude's.

Fracture City

Steve Cushman

I wasn't normally a smoker but that night when Rothco, the ER charge nurse, joined me outside and offered me a cigarette I gladly took it. I had just X-rayed my first dead person, a twelve-year-old with a thin line of peach fuzz across his upper lip. We didn't normally have to X-ray dead people, but the morgue's machine was broken so they'd called and asked if we'd shoot some films, see if he had any fractures to go along with the bleeding in his brain that had killed him. The story I'd heard was that he'd been walking home when a car hit him. What he was doing on the side of the road in the dark didn't seem to matter.

After finishing the X-rays, a little after midnight, I had walked out the side door of the hospital. It didn't make sense to me that the night was so alive with the sound of cicadas and frogs when inside, no more than thirty yards away, this boy was lying dead on a stretcher. I wondered what his parents were doing, and if they had any idea their son wasn't home. Maybe they were already on their way to the hospital. I wondered what my mother was doing—probably sleeping—and if she was dreaming about me. If she did dream about me was it twelve-year-old me or the current 23-year-old version? Was I the same person to her, never changing?

This was all rolling around in my mind when I saw Rothco walk out of the hospital and come towards me. He was in his forties, shaved his head and rarely smiled.

I took the cigarette he offered, puffed on it twice and tried not to cough.

He lit his own, then said, 'Sorry to make you X-ray that kid back there.'

'It's part of the job,' I said. 'People die every day.'

He raised his eyebrows and nodded as if to say, *Sure, try to be tough.* After exhaling a wall of smoke, he said, 'My mother is dying.'

'Sorry.'

'Pancreatic cancer. Every morning when I get home, I expect to find her dead.'

This was the most he'd ever spoken to me. I wondered if he'd seen me almost lose it in there, when I had to lift the kid's leg and set it on an X-ray cassette—how I had to wipe my face to keep from crying. If this was his attempt to comfort me in some way.

'I moved in with her and switched to night shift three months ago when she got sick,' he said. 'This way I'm with her during the day, and she's sleeping when I'm at work.'

Across the road, a pair of bats circled a streetlight, consuming bugs, completely in control of their flight. I didn't feel in control of anything.

'Sometimes I check on her on my lunchbreak,' Rothco said, 'just to make sure she's breathing.'

'I'm sorry,' I said. I'd whispered the same words to the dead boy when the two of us were alone in the trauma room.

Cars drove by on the road, their speed and the darkness making it hard to tell their make and model, sometimes even their color. Around the corner from us, a woman was talking on a cell phone, telling someone that her baby had a fever.

Rothco took a final drag of his cigarette, tossed it on the ground and stomped it out. 'I'm going to ride over there now, check on her. You want to come? Twenty minutes round trip.'

More cars pulled into the ER parking lot, and I wondered if one of them might be driven by the kid's parents. I imagined them breaking down when they saw their boy. His face was bruised but not too bad. What they wouldn't be able to see was the hemorrhage in his brain, and how both of his femurs and his pelvis were fractured.

'Yeah,' I said, 'I'll go.' I'd told Ray, the other X-ray tech, that I just needed to get some air, but I'd deal with him when I got back, say I'd decided to go ahead and take my break.

When Rothco turned the key of his truck, Johnny Cash boomed from the door panels. We drove through the neighborhood that bordered the hospital, heading in the opposite direction of the apartment I'd moved into three months ago after finishing X-ray school, leaving my mother in our house by herself. I'd moved out because I had a real job and could afford it and I was an adult; it was time to go. But now, I felt guilty for leaving her. My father had been gone for over a decade, and my sister had moved to North Carolina two years ago.

'You know,' Rothco said, 'if you're going to stay in this game a long time you'll see a lot worse than that kid. You'll see babies with limbs missing, burn marks on their foreheads. You'll see shit you won't ever forget. Some nights, I swear, it's like fracture city in there.'

'Great,' I said.

'You could always go work at McDonald's, or the mall.' I knew he was joking, but I didn't laugh; it wasn't funny. None of this was.

We didn't speak again until we pulled into his mother's crushed-stone driveway. The house was white and square, much bigger than the one I'd grown up in. There was a row of palm trees in the front yard by the road, and a wooden fence circled the back yard.

Rothco climbed out and shut his door, then opened it again. 'You coming?'

The inside of the house was sparse, and Rothco didn't turn on the lights, so I could barely make out a couch, a love seat and a recliner. Was this what it was like to be a burglar, to be able to see only the outlines of what was in front and around you?

Rothco said, 'I'll be right back,' then turned down the main hall leading away from where I stood.

I opened the sliding glass doors that led to the back yard. There was no grass, only a pool surrounded by cement. With the underwater lights on, I could see the steps at the shallow end. I sat on one of the lounge chairs and listened to the hum of the AC. I thought again of my mother. Three days ago, she'd left a message on my answering machine, asking if I could come over and help her get the lawnmower started. She said she thought it might be the spark plug or maybe she'd flooded it. I stood there and listened to her leave the message and didn't pick up the phone or call her back because I didn't want to mow that damn yard I'd mowed thousands of times before. Now, sitting by the pool, I wished I'd driven over to her house right then or the next morning, and replaced the blade and checked the spark plug and gone ahead and mowed the yard.

'Want a beer?' Rothco was standing at the door, holding two bottles of Miller Lite.

I took the one he offered. He sat in the chair opposite me, put his cell phone and keys on the ground between us and took a long swallow from his beer.

'She okay?' I asked.

'She's alive. I don't know how much longer she'll last—maybe a week or two. Pancreatic cancer is a bitch.'

'Do you like being a nurse?' I hadn't known I was going to ask the question until the words left my lips, but now I'd said them his answer seemed important.

'Sure, it's a job. Sometimes you even get to help people. What about you? You like being an X-ray tech?'

'I guess,' I said.

If you'd asked me when I graduated from high school what my future plans were, I can guarantee you that becoming an X-ray tech wasn't one of them. But three years ago, when I was still stocking shelves at Target and complaining every night about how the job had no future, my mother showed me an article in the Sunday paper about careers in radiology. The article promised indoor work, steady employment, decent pay, and the opportunity to work with doctors and nurses. Nowhere did it mention you might have to X-ray dead people. Still, overall, I did like my job.

We finished our beers in silence, then Rothco stood up and announced he had to take a piss. He wasn't gone five seconds before I picked up his cell phone and dialed my mother's landline. I knew she kept an old yellow rotary phone on her nightstand, and as it rang two, three times, I imagined her stirring in her sleep, wondering if what she was hearing was real or imagined, part of the dream she was wrapped up in.

It rang four, five times. I needed her to pick up. I didn't know what I'd say, wasn't even sure I would be able to speak. I could see her brown-gray hair draped over her face and her sleepy eyes. And although I felt guilty for waking her up and possibly ruining a good dream, that guilt was nothing compared to the need I had to hear her voice; I needed to know she was alive, and when I drove over to her house in the morning with donuts and coffee she would be there to receive me.

There was a soft click, the sound of pillows shuffling, followed by a voice, my mother's, faint and tired. 'Hello, yes.'

I hung up without a word, let out a big breath and lowered my head into my hands.

A couple minutes later, Rothco opened the sliding doors, ran past me still dressed in his green hospital scrubs, and dove into the pool; a spray of water hit against the fence. 'Come on in,' he said after he surfaced, laughing. 'It'll wake you up, help you get through the rest of the night.'

I didn't have any other clothes, but I could get more scrubs at the hospital. That wasn't really a problem. I'd held a dead boy's leg; I'd heard my mother's voice. And I knew that in a half-hour I'd be back at work X-raying more patients. I stood up and eyed the water, the lights below the surface turning everything an easy blue. I held my breath and ran with everything I had into the pool's open arms.

My Mother, the Gardenia

Darci Flatley

When Mom dies, she wants every viable organ to be donated to those in need. Not only her heart and kidneys, but she also wants her skin donated to burn victims, her cataracts to the blind. And she doesn't want a prolonged death. If she can't get around without the aid of a machine, she wants the cords unplugged. She's frequently told me to smother her if taking her off a ventilator isn't an option.

After the donations, she wants to be cremated. But she doesn't want to end up in a decorated urn on a mantelpiece; she wants her ashes to be turned into this biodegradable tree planter she read about—a pretty magnolia, or one of the trees that turns a fiery orange in the fall. She wants a Catholic funeral, because she holds on to the tradition of the Church she grew up in, but just a simple prayer as we plant her tree. Maybe a few words.

'And don't you dare plant me back up in Pennsylvania,' she says. 'Plant me somewhere the three of you kids can all visit.'

~

Mom moved to Florida from Pennsylvania with her best friend, Cindy, when they were twenty-three. They didn't have jobs lined up or housing secured. They didn't know anyone in Florida either. But they could live together in Cocoa Beach and get away from the overcast, dreary town of their childhood.

Mom packed her car with her clothes, some books and photos, and went to pick up Cindy. The two found a good radio station and started the fourteen-hour drive along the East Coast. I imagine them like Thelma and Louise: sunglasses on, windows down and hair blowing all over the place. Music blasting as they sing, loudly and out of tune, to each other, sipping on sodas and passing Twizzlers back and forth. I can see them cheering, hooting and hollering, as they cross the border from Georgia into Florida. They pull the car over and take a photo in front of the *Welcome to Florida!* sign, big blocky sunglasses falling off Cindy's nose and a bandana holding Mom's hair back. In the welcome center, they indulge in the free freshly squeezed orange juice and take a quick bathroom break. 'Let's go!' Mom yells to Cindy. 'We've still got six hours ahead of us.'

~

I have Mom's laugh—loud, demanding of attention. I have her height. I have her metabolism. I have her tendency to cry easily, although she says this comes from her mom. I also have her back.

She had to have an intense surgery to fix it. 'Her vertebrae aren't aligned,' her surgeon explained to me. 'Instead, they look like a set of stairs.'

In late January, Mom and I drove to the hospital for a four-hour surgery. During intake, I signed paperwork that made me her power of attorney. In case surgery didn't go as planned, I was to make the decisions on what would happen next. We giggled as we talked about teas I could pour down her throat that would kill her if she ended up paralyzed, but that would also make her death look natural so I wouldn't go to jail. We didn't believe anything could go wrong.

Four hours into the surgery, a nurse told me about a complication the surgeons had found: Mom's nerves had rooted themselves into a cyst. When I'd signed her in, I hadn't spent time thinking about if things didn't run smoothly. I'd never really considered complications.

~

Whenever Dad and I argued, he would end his side of the fight with the same insult: 'You're just like your mother.' He'd make sure the words stung, emphasizing *your mother*. But I have Dad's nose. I have his complexion. I have his bone structure. I have his hair, too; I wonder if he started to gray in his early twenties. I have his stubbornness.

'You're just like your mother.' He planted this idea in my head at a young age. He watered it and watched it grow as his dislike of Mom led to a resentment of me.

~

Gardenia bushes are hardy plants. They're extremely aromatic too. They bloom twice a year: once in early spring and again in midsummer. Big, fluffy white flowers find their place within the shiny deep-green leaves.

Our neighbor had a row of gardenias between his property line and the road. Once the flowers had bloomed each year, Mom would slow our car down and lower the windows so my siblings and I could stick our hands out and try to pluck them as we drove past. We'd end up with a bushel each by the time we reached our driveway.

We had about three or four gardenia bushes throughout our own property. I used to fill out my bouquets with flowers picked from them.

Mom would put the gardenias in three vases; she'd keep one in the kitchen, one on her nightstand, and one on the dining table. We'd picked the flowers for her, after all.

~

I wasn't sure how entangled Mom's nervous system was with the cyst, but I knew she wouldn't want any pain. I told the doctors to remove it even though it could leave her paralyzed.

As they left to finish the operation, I tried to imagine Mom's spine. I could see the stairs of her vertebrae with her nervous system winding around them like vines. I remembered pictures of cysts I'd seen in a science class; I imagined the bulb of it hiding in the vines of her nerves, its own roots weaving and knotting it further into her pain receptors.

I wondered if I'd made the right decision. What if Mom was paralyzed? I knew she'd never want a life like that. Could I give her the support she needed, knowing it was my fault she was in this state? Or, worst-case scenario, could I actually go through with euthanizing my own mother?

I pictured a surgeon trimming away at the cyst with his scalpel, then tracing its roots and mixing them up with the vines of her nerves. He could so easily slice through the wrong branch.

~

Cindy and Mom didn't live together for too long. Cindy's boyfriend began to steal Mom's rent money and use it to buy drugs. The day a piece of her grandmother's jewelry disappeared, she moved out.

She didn't go back to Pennsylvania, though; she had begun to make connections in Florida and needed to cultivate them. She moved into a pink boarding house right across the street from the Intercoastal Waterway, a river that flows between the beaches of the Atlantic and the coastline of Florida. 'I could see your father from my window,' she's often told me. 'He liked to eat his breakfast outside. I watched him change the oil in his car, read the newspaper, drink some coffee.' Mom always starts to laugh after telling me about the man she met. 'He did everything for himself, and then we got married.'

~

I wasn't a good baby. I needed to be held at all times, and not just by anyone—I needed to be held by Mom. Because of this, she learned how to do everything one-handed. There are countless photos of her cooking with me on her hip. Of her playing with Evan, my older brother, while I'm in her lap. Of her cradling my baby sister Emily in one arm while hugging me close to her leg with the other.

I've never grown out of needing to be held. I hug my mom every time I see her and every time I leave her. Mom's arms always feel the same. She holds me tight and close. Because she's a few inches taller than I am, my nose nestles into her neck, and I can smell her perfume—it reminds me of clean linen candles and gardenias. She kisses the soft spot behind my ear and laughs as she tells me how much she loves me.

~

After Mom's surgery, a nurse told me I was allowed access to the room they were about to move her into. Her face was swollen because she'd been lying on it for eight hours, and she was in obvious pain. I backed into a corner of the room to try to get out of the nurses' way as they attached wires and tubes to Mom, making me wonder how I was going to hug her.

She answered their questions through gritted teeth, then sighed with relief when the room cleared out and the morphine started to work. 'Come here, doodlebug,' she whispered to me.

I hadn't moved from the corner and was just staring at this broken image of my mom. I crept over to her bedside and leaned down to give her a hug. Her arms held me as tight as they always had.

~

Gardenias like acidic earth; potting soil will kill them on its own, but the addition of used coffee grounds will provide the needed acidity. They are also picky about water: they practically like to be drowned, but not too often or their roots will begin to rot, and the soil can't dry out or their branches will become brittle enough to break. They're prone to insects; tiny millipede-like bugs will eat through their leaves. Ideal exposure to sunlight is difficult to gauge as well—too much and the leaves turn yellow and drop, too little and they shrivel.

But these plants are resilient.

~

Four days after her surgery, Mom was supposed to come home with me. Instead, a social worker walked into her hospital room and asked to speak with her power of attorney.

I followed the social worker outside. 'We can't send your mom home just yet,' she said. 'She needs more intensive rehab in order to get her walking again.' She handed me a list of nursing homes and rehabilitation centers. 'I'll come see you in a few hours once you've figured out where to move her.'

I watched the social worker walk away before going back into Mom's room. She had been sleeping for most of the day. Each morning, a nurse would force her out of bed, strap her into a harness to prevent falls, and get her to walk a lap through the corridors. It took everything out of her.

In telling the doctors to cut the cyst out of Mom's spine, I had given them permission to paralyze her from the knee down in her left leg. Her stability was gone. Her balance was off. The slightest breeze, and she could come crashing to the ground. If your mom is paralyzed and you're not there to catch her if she falls, is that your fault?

~

We learned how to fight from our parents. We knew that arguments aren't supposed to be quiet—you have to yell and scream and throw your hands up in the air. You only ever get quiet when you really want to hurt someone. We learned how to manipulate each other. We learned how to hold a grudge for years.

~

More people than Dad have told me I am just like my mother—more people than I can think of, from other family members, to my parents' coworkers and friends, to strangers who catch us joking with each other in check-out lines. It's easy to see.

The first time I realized I was my mother's daughter, the two of us were in a Winn-Dixie supermarket. I tagged along with Mom like I usually did because I liked to be around her; I liked the one-on-one time it gave us, and the privacy it allowed for me to tell her things I didn't want my siblings to overhear.

Mom asked me to run an aisle over and grab something she had missed. When I was walking back, I got distracted by something on the shelves. Soon I was reading the boxes and scanning the cans of soup while dancing to the music that played over the speakers. When I snapped out of it, I turned to see Mom doing the exact same thing at the other end of the aisle. I was mortified, but couldn't wait to tell her. 'You really are mine,' she said in response. We giggled at the coincidence and finished collecting the items on the list.

Many of Mom's qualities and traits and habits have always been present in me. Growing up I was mostly unaware of them, but I've realized how deeply they are within me.

~

I thought I would be discussing engagement with a serious boyfriend. I thought I would be looking at prospective high-paying jobs. I thought I would have my mom, in perfect health, forever.

Instead, I was lifting her out of her wheelchair and into the front seat of my car. I was buckling her in because she couldn't do so herself. I was adjusting and readjusting the seat to find a comfortable position for her. I was signing paperwork at the nursing home she would be living in until she could climb stairs again. I was taking a semester off from college, paying the bills, and visiting Mom every day.

I was begging my older brother to come down to help me. I was begging my little sister to visit Mom after she was done with school. I was sobbing on the phone to my friends from college. I was updating family members. I was politely telling friends that Mom wasn't ready for visitors.

I was assembling a walker and lifted toilet seat for when Mom came home. I was removing the box-spring to lower her mattress so it would be easier for her to get into bed. I was moving the furniture around so she'd have access to the house with her walker. I was tightening the railing along the stairs. I was moving rugs into the closets. I was installing a baby gate to keep the dogs from tripping Mom.

I was phoning the insurance company and medical staff every day to get Mom out of the nursing home she was in. I was yelling at nurses for being neglectful, after I found out she'd waited hours for assistance to use the restroom. I was demanding that her physical therapist help her learn to climb four stairs before he helped her do anything else so I could bring her home.

There were a lot of things I'd got wrong about what my life would be like at twenty.

~

'I can't believe you're moving to California at twenty-three,' Mom said. 'I could never be that brave.'

She was sitting on my bed and keeping me company while I tried to pack up my entire life in three suitcases. 'But didn't you move to Florida when you were my age?' I asked.

'I had just finished my associate degree and had been working at the day care for a while. I was about twenty-three, so I guess you're right, yeah.'

'I guess I get the bravery from you, then,' I told her.

~

After moving to California, I accidentally started to garden. The state was too brown; I missed the lush greenery of Florida. I began with a spider plant—something Mimi, Mom's mom, had grown for years with ease. I called Mimi to ask what she did to keep them thriving, and she gave me a few tips that I've since learned apply to most house plants.

The spider plant I purchased is all green, although they usually have a white stripe down each leaf. I put the plant in a macramé hanger so its leaves could grow freely, like Mimi had said to do. Ever since then, every few days I dip a fingertip into the soil, searching for moisture. If I can't find any, I give the plant a drink and breathe in the smell of wet dirt.

~

I'd woken up early on the day Mom was finally able to come home after her surgery. I cleaned the entire house and bathed the dogs. I made sure there wasn't anything that could cause her to fall.

For the millionth time I walked outside to make sure the stairs were secure, and I noticed the gardenias had bloomed. I gathered some, placed them in three vases, and set one in the kitchen, one on her nightstand, and one on the dining table. They were always for her.

~

After propagating my spider plant a few times and adding a couple new plant varieties to my collection, I noticed I was missing a plant that demanded space. I walked into my local nursery to find a larger plant to put in an empty corner of my bedroom—I wanted either a fiddle-leaf fig or a monstera.

I turned the corner and was hit with the sweet, light smell of gardenias. I realized I wasn't missing a plant demanding of space, but a plant that felt like home.

After shifting through the five or six bushes in the nursery, I found the one with the smallest girth. I picked out a large terracotta planter, threw a bag of acidic soil over my shoulder and made my way to the front to pay for the plant that smelled like Mom.

Transcendental Numbers

C.A. Limina

He couldn't finish a high school trigonometry question, this time. I barely passed any of my math classes, but even I can see the steps he failed to take on the first try. All the numbers he once jotted on his arms with Sharpies, the formulas he once taught in front of MIT students, the gratuitously complex equations he once threw at me every afternoon on the drive home—gone. Devoured. After the next radiotherapy session, I'll be teaching my husband how to count.

'Come on, Herman.' I slap the notebook back onto his food table, pushing aside plates of vomit-hued Jell-O and dried apple slices. 'You snore out problems harder than this. What, now that I'm asking for one of your overly elaborate presentations, you chicken out? Pathetic.'

Herman looks at me then, his eyes like a meadow filled with yellow flowers. Pale gold, as F. Scott Fitzgerald would've said. Even before the diagnosis Herman wouldn't have known anything about Fitzgerald, but back then I would've told him anyway. Showing off useless knowledge was our means of flirting. If he recited pi to the ten-thousandth digit, I would quote the entirety of Othello in return. That was how we loved. That was how we were.

He can't recite pi to the ten-thousandth digit anymore.

The doctor comes in, and I count the four times she looks at her silver-plated watch, as if she's waiting for the end to come. 'He has an estimated three months to live,' she tells me, and I haven't seen a performance as atrocious since Herman made me sit through an Adam Sandler movie. 'There are other experimental treatments you might want to try, but none of them are guaranteed to work. There is one study, though, that seems promising—'

'As promising as the last one was, Dr Winchell?' I ask. 'As promising as the other snake oils you've tossed our way? What, will this one give him five, six more days to live?'

She falls silent, and Herman's shrivelled fingers clutch mine. 'George,' he whispers, 'be polite. She's—she's trying to help.'

I can feel the coughs he was holding back, the tremors running down his fingers to mine. I imagine the sun setting on the horizon in his eyes, dissolving as the rest of his face grays. Petals. Rose petals and rain. It'll be an open casket funeral, and I'll be there, weeping equations only he could've solved.

~

Three nights later, Dr Winchell tells us Herman is well enough to make a coffin out of our bedroom. I gather the notebooks, the pill bottles, the IV fluids and the rest of our medical paraphernalia, then wheel Herman into our car. The sedan wheezes as we move out of the hospital parking lot, hacking harder than Herman ever would in front of me. Death and disinfectant stick to my turtleneck, and I know no matter how many times I run it through the washing machine, I'll still wake up at three in the morning, scrubbing the smell from my skin. I'll never remember Herman for the pasture in his eyes, or the taste of tangerines on his lips during our wedding day—only the pungency of iodoform ripping through aged cashmere.

'George,' Herman chokes out, 'have I ever told you about transcendental numbers?'

There are white holes poked into the night. The town sleeps, uneasy but tranquil, the traffic lights flickering from green to red in the distance. Only one other car drives through, but we wait for a solid two minutes.

'No,' I lie to him. I look at him, expectant. 'What are they?'

He tells me everything I already knew from the hospital nights. His descriptions have grown blander. The first night at the hospital, they were the irrationality of the universe, the absurdity of life. By the fourth night, they had devolved into numbers that go on, and on, and on, and aren't countable for some reason. Tonight, he looks back at me, the desperation in his furrowed brows evident. 'I—I can't remember,' he whispers. 'But it's important. I know it's important.'

The light is green. I stare at him, still, until the light turns red again. Nobody honks behind me.

'Pi,' I say. I look back at the road. 'One of them is pi. You told me, once.'

There's the comic warmth of a cartoon light bulb hanging over his head, and he laughs. 'Yes. Pi. One of the most famous transcendental numbers in history,' he lectures. 'It's ridiculous, I know, but I truly do believe that memorizing pi is the key to understanding the cosmos. Every single digit, running across the pages, they all mean something. There's a digit for the Big Bang. There's a digit for the formation of Earth. There's a digit for every philosopher, for every war, for every story and artist caught in time. There's a digit for me. There's a digit for you.' He pauses. 'And there's a digit for miracles, too.'

Miracles.

All at once, memories of my father's leather Bible and the mascara streaking down my mother's cheeks strike my mind. Miracles were all they talked about in those days. The same miracle that had saved my uncle from his drunken stupors took my older sister to heaven before I turned thirteen. I remember the coughing, the hospital trip, the phone call at three in the morning. *She's gone, sir.* It was the only time I saw my father cry.

When I fell from an apple tree on my fifteenth birthday, a failed attempt to escape a party, my parents had never driven faster than they did then, swerving past trucks and buses to the hospital. And for what? A sprained ankle. *Thank God*, they whispered in their embrace, suffocating me on the hospital bed. *Oh, thank God you're all right.* Most days, I fooled myself into thinking they were wholly concerned for me. But their grasps told the story; their hands glided over the back of my neck, feeling for long strands of blonde hair that weren't there, pretending they were hugging a girl who was six feet in the dirt. A resurrection had occurred in their heads, a form of salvation.

I don't believe in miracles—not now, not then. Life is a book written by a hack, and the plot threads are always the same. I knew it was too late for my father when my mother called during my college course, and I knew it was too late for my mother when she didn't leave any letters by my flat door for Christmas. It was always the same song and dance: the coughing, the hospital, the call at 3 a.m. My parents sought miracles; I only ask for peaceful conclusions.

Then I remember the years before Herman and I got married.

'It's never going to happen,' I'd told him in this very car, shaking my head. 'These nutcases are talking about making a wall and throwing homosexuals behind it so we all starve to death—they're not going to legalize our union.'

'It's in pi, George,' Herman said, when he still had a head of golden hair. 'It'll happen. You need to see the glass is half full.'

'How about you tell that to your MIT mates and see how well it goes,' I spat back. 'And what happens in pi—God knows how you know it does—doesn't necessarily happen here, and if it does, it probably won't happen while we're alive. Don't go Nostradamus on me, Herman. I'm not keen on dating an idiot.'

He laughed, shaking his head. 'You'll see. The statistics are there. People are coming around.'

I remember stopping the car, at one point, and feeling the familiar bite of optimism. I'd forgotten the song and dance, the beat of the universe pounding under our feet. Perhaps my parents were right. Perhaps.

I shook my head. 'They're not coming around fast enough.'

That was sixteen years ago. I know, because he used to tell me after our clock struck twelve in the evening, when we both stopped pretending to be asleep in each other's arms. 'Sixteen years of marriage,' he'd start, 'twenty years of being together. Twenty-eight years of being a pretentious knob. An infinity, stretching out to the future.' Then he'd drift off, pillow talking the only way he knew how: by reciting pi. 'Three point one four one five nine two six …'

Perhaps it was the ease of his hand as he dragged lines onto a chalkboard. Maybe it was the way he'd scribble out half-baked solutions to unknown questions on napkins when we went out for coffee. More likely, it's the rhythm of his heart beating in his chest when we fall asleep, echoing from the cushions and duvet. Regardless, I'd like to think in a world without miracles, Herman comes the closest to being one.

~

The book in my lap feels heavier by the minute. Herman lies on our bed before me with his unblinking eyes and open mouth, murmuring nothings in a half-dream. Sirens and headlights blare past the blinds, and I struggle to remember how I got here.

'Do you need a glass of water?' I ask.

His gaze moves up to me. 'No. No, thank you, darling George.' He huffs. 'Could you repeat what you said? About the kids on the island. I'm sorry, sweetheart, it's slipped my mind.'

I don't want him to die. I glance down at William Golding's prose in my lap, and I close the book, chiding yet soothing my psyche. I need him to live. I need him to be alive. And I don't want him to die.

'Let's change the pace a bit,' I say. I walk across the room to grab my laptop from my work desk, opening it as I walk back to the bed. 'Have something more on your level.'

Herman stares in curiosity as I type in numbers.

'I'm hoping you remember this better than I'll be able to read it,' I say with a chuckle.

The stiffness of his form suggests expectation, anticipation, perhaps even a thrill, but it takes me a moment to register this as positive.

'Three,' I exhale in prayer. Even in his deterioration, he smiles, greeting the numbers that come next. 'Point one four …'

~

From then on, each night I read out the digits of pi from the light of my laptop, usually not even getting to the hundredth before Herman drifts off to sleep. I don't mind. The numbers are etched into my brain: 3.1415926535 …

It makes no sense to me, but I know it does to him. It's always made sense to him, even if there's not much of him left. It's never just numbers, with him around.

~

Eight months later, he's still alive, though only barely. His conditions worsened, so I had him moved back into the hospital. Tonight he blinks once, twice, the pasture in his eyes now the Russian taiga, ravaged by winter winds. I've been made to use a diaper on him, and feed him regularly, like a child. A child of numbers.

I read out to him, 'Three point one four one five nine two six five three five …'

A normal evening. But the atmosphere is different. The numbers aren't the same as they were before; they're heavier, now.

I look down at his bed. He's staring up at me, his eyes wide with fear. The oxygen monitor screams like a high school girl in a horror movie, and I realize that he's coughing. He's coughing, in front of me.

'Don't you dare,' is all I can say. I throw the laptop aside and grab on to him, mouthing 'don't you dare' at various volumes. He's still looking at me, his eyes glossing over, and panic swells in my veins. 'Don't you dare leave me, Herman. Don't you dare leave me here.'

But all my words fail. The numbers have hijacked their meaning.

'We can still do this,' I tell him, because all my cynicism has failed me, all my cautions have betrayed me, none of my words matter anymore. 'There's still a digit of miracles. It's still there. We'll look together, you and I. Just—just—'

He wheezes. He breathes, but no oxygen gets in. Years of ache.

'Three,' I spit out finally, unable to say anything else after all this time, 'point one four one five nine two six five—'

He wheezes again, hacking. The nurse comes by; she's screaming for others to assist. The numbers are the only things that matter now.

'Three five—'

His hands reach out, caressing my face.

'Eight … eight …' My eyes sting. 'Nine—'

His wheezing stops. His face goes blank.

I clutch his fingers, even as the nurses pull me away. 'Seven nine …' My vision is blurry as I repeat myself. 'Seven nine … six …'

Time stops. Nothing changes.

The digits hold no miracle, and yet his eyes are still open. The sun has yet to set on the meadow.

'Three,' he whispers.

I pause.

'It's … it's three.' He breathes in. This time, he only feels relief. 'Not six.'

And the numbers don't matter anymore.

Not Done with All That

Jann Everard

The light is hazy, low winter sun through sheer curtains. Two La-Z-Boy recliners sit empty and sagging on shaggy brown carpet.

'Where are your roommates?' Ann asks. She pulls at a brass button that dangles from the pocket of her jeans. The single thread that holds the button breaks.

Will's gaze drops to her knees. 'At the library,' he says.

She makes the first move, drawing him down to the carpet to sit astride his hips. It doesn't take long before they both shudder and cry out. She slides next to him and turns her cheek to the carpet's rough fibres.

His hand brushes her thigh. 'Annie?'

She wants him to initiate more, to feel the hard eagerness of her breasts. 'What do you like about me?' she asks.

He leans forward. Through the thin Indian gauze of her shirt, she feels teeth graze her nipple. 'What's not to like?'

~

Against Ann's closed eyelids, morning sunlight glows red and gold. She presses into the foam mattress, the flatness of her chest still a surprise. Cheap sheets, bought in a needless moment of thrift, scratch her skin and evoke again Will's raspy carpet. It must be the sleeping pills she's taking; her dreams are all from the past.

Swinging her legs over the side of the bed, she reaches for her glasses, then stretches upright. She has been declared 'cancer free'—free to carry on and to live normally. She circles her hips left, then right, sensing a brightness in her pelvis, an elasticity that's been absent for some time, until this morning's dream. She feels more positive than she's felt in weeks.

Down the hall, the spare bedroom door is closed, but the light is on. It creates a yellow strip on the floorboards that catches her eye. So, Martin is up. He's become an early bird, often showered and shaved long before she wakes.

The bathroom door is ajar, her husband's face reflected in the mirror above the sink. She hesitates, needing badly to relieve her full bladder. In the past, she would have joined him in the bathroom, unembarrassed to strip or pee in front of him as he stroked the razor over his skin, to take a moment to enjoy his naked body, confident that he enjoyed her nakedness too. But these days, she is unsure of the rules.

'Morning,' she calls.

'I'll be out in a sec,' he answers.

The damp heat of the bathroom washes over her as he opens the door and gives her a peck on the cheek. The kiss is spare and dutiful, and her earlier positivity seeps away. She slumps against the wall.

'You didn't sleep well?' he asks.

'I slept fine. How about you?'

He won't meet her eyes. 'Did you have to take anything for the pain?'

'I'm fine. Are you okay?'

His smile is forced, his nod too jaunty. She reaches out to rub a speck of shaving lotion off his jawbone. But he jerks back, glancing towards then away from her pajama top where it lies flat against her chest. Dropping her hand, she crosses her arms and rubs her shoulders, pretending to be cold.

'Are the kids coming home this weekend?' he asks, red-faced now, and restless.

'They're driving down on Friday. Should be here for supper.'

He nods. 'That'll be nice. Some company for you.'

She's about to point out that he is company, too, but instead says, 'I have to go,' and shrugs towards the bathroom. He twists away, giving her ample room to get by.

Behind the closed door, she runs the bath, turning the hot water to full so that the mirror steams and reflects nothing. She adds bubbles from the pink bottle that stands next to the pink soap and the pink hairbrush—all well-meaning gifts. When she's immersed in the tub, her small belly bobs above the waterline as her breasts once did. It stirs another memory from when she was a student, this time of Will carving a bar of Ivory soap into the hourglass shape of a woman's body. While they were in the bath together, he'd lathered her leg then scraped his razor over the creamy foam in long sweeps. The bar had floated on the scummy water: two proud cones, the nipples tipped with her coral nail polish.

She glances down at her scars to push away the mental images. It's time to face the day. And reality. It's time to be forward thinking. To use positive self-talk.

She shaves her legs and underarms, tweezes a few stray hairs from her inner thigh, another that has sprouted near her navel. She will not let herself go. She will 'Look Good, Feel Better', just as the ladies at the workshop advised. She will be encouraged by the social workers who write in their pamphlets that 'issues of sexuality with your partner are common and can be worked through'.

In all their years of marriage, Martin has never shared the bath with her. 'It's too small, too awkward to incite intimacies,' he complained. He always preferred the bedroom, where he would approach her from behind, cupping her breasts as she brushed her hair before the closet mirror. Martin was first to notice the lump. Martin, who has been her confidant, her partner in all things; who is father to her children. If she had been more vigilant, her cancer might have been discovered earlier, the need for a double mastectomy avoided. Martin might still be sleeping with her in the master bedroom. He has not touched her intimately since the surgery.

She tries to hold back, tries to make this the first tear-free day since her diagnosis, but gives up. So many stressful weeks have gone by. On which night, disrupted by her worry or pain, did Martin move to the spare bedroom? She'd encouraged it, anxious that he not suffer because of her sleeplessness. But the arrangement, intended to be temporary, now seems permanent.

Not long ago, she read a novel featuring a married couple. Years into their marriage, the wife told the husband that, from that day, everything would stay the same except she was 'done with all that'. In the story, things did stay the same, except the man slept with a neighbouring widow instead of his wife. That wasn't the important part of the story, not the main plot. But Ann still wonders, long after she returned the book to the library: without sex, how could things possibly stay the same between the man and his wife?

~

'I'll be late tonight. We're hammering out a contract with the city. I don't know what my schedule will be like for a while.' Martin pours coffee from the enamel carafe Ann likes them to use at the breakfast table. He hands her the creamer, reaching for his cell phone as if to give authority to his words.

She pads barefoot to the far side of the kitchen, removes a spoon from the drawer and taps it against her palm. Has he forgotten that he promised to be free tonight? Not promised exactly, but she'd asked him whether he had plans and thought it was clear she wanted him to set them aside. 'I hoped we'd trim the forsythia back this evening. And plant the annuals. Have the chance to catch up on things.'

Again, he gazes past her. 'I know we're late getting the plants in,' he says.

She's unsure whether he's missed her intended message or is avoiding it. They need to talk now that the immediate crisis is over, her surgery successful, life moving on. The social worker suggested a quiet evening together doing something they enjoy. 'If your partner is not a great talker,' she said, 'sometimes you have to do it yourself. Talk, talk, talk—he may not talk back, but he'll be listening.'

Martin sighs. 'I'm sorry. There's so much going on at work that I need to be on top of. I think you should hire someone to help with the garden.'

She stares out the kitchen window at a tulip, perfectly formed, sexually red. Does she dare ask him, right at this moment, whether she is still attractive to him, whether it would help if she had breast reconstruction surgery, how he feels about false breasts? Does the idea of implants repulse him more than no breasts at all? It took ten months after each of the boys stopped nursing before he reclaimed her nipples.

'I have an appointment with the surgeon tomorrow,' she says.

As she waits, the coffee grows cold in her hand. He doesn't ask whether he should join her. He squeezes her shoulder as he leaves the kitchen. Moments later, the automatic garage door makes its usual grating sound six inches before it snugs up against the roof. The digital clock is silent as the readout changes from 7.45 to 7.46.

~

She moves to her desk in the kitchen nook. Her phone beckons with its beeps and reminders from her calendar: tomorrow's consultation, a follow-up with her GP in three weeks. She could cancel the appointment with the surgeon, but what would she say to the receptionist? *There is no need to reconstruct my breasts. There is no foundation on which to attach them.* She puts the phone back down.

Coffee mug in hand, she wanders the house. It's tidy, the laundry done, the breakfast dishes set to clean in the stainless-steel washer that reminds her of a hospital sterilizer. She stands at the door of the master bedroom staring at the queen-sized bed, linens disrupted on only one side. One quick hike and the duvet settles into place, then she is down the hall, avoiding the spare bedroom and whatever secret sourness it might hold.

Her computer glows to life. During the first awful days after she learned she had cancer, she signed up with Facebook. It made a good distraction to contact people from her past; they knew nothing about her illness. They shared the titles of good books, pictures of their grown children, funny videos that had gone viral—nothing personal.

Today there's a friend request from a Belgian girl whom Ann has not heard from since eleventh grade. Jeannine Charlier's parents were journalists, and after only three years in the country they moved on to their next assignment. With her European clothes and hybrid accent of English and French, Jeannine had been one of Ann's favourite friends.

Almost as soon as she accepts Jeannine's request, a message arrives: *Annie, my old friend, there is someone who wants to talk to you.*

Although the message is odd, Ann replies that she is looking forward to talking.

Minutes later, a request appears from Denis Dumont. She stares at the thumbnail, unsure. From Jeannine comes a new message: *You remember my brother's friend Denis? You two had such a nice time together. He asks after you. You must be nice to him. He has had a heart transplant but is much better now.*

Denis. Until now, she hadn't known his last name. He'd visited Jeannine's family for a week when Ann was seventeen, and they spent evenings together in the Charlier family's basement, kissing until their lips were sore. Only a week of innocent, teenage making out, and he was asking after her?

She types: Jeannine, *I'm flattered that he remembers me, but why do you think he wants to be in touch now?*

The answer is swift: *He says he only wants to connect with people who knew his real heart. Will you be able to write to him in French?*

His real heart? She suspects the expression has suffered in translation, but her French is not good enough to be sure.

~

Edging the garden calms her, with the slight resistance of the lawn to the blade before she pushes on the tool with the ball of her foot, the clean slice, the scruff of grass and weed tossed aside.

Jeannine's message still puzzles her. It suggests that Denis understandably feels different since his transplant, but also disassociated from his new heart. Their situations are very different, but is it possible she could feel that ambivalence to reconstructed breasts? Or perhaps it is not Denis but his relationships that have changed, his experience showing him his real friends. A conversation with him could be interesting; she could use an objective male perspective. But it is out of the question. He is a stranger, not someone she can talk to on such a personal level.

The next push on the edger tweaks a muscle; pain shoots

through her shoulder. She pulls off her work gloves and throws them towards the potting shed. They lie in the grass, yellow like a nearby dandelion.

'Fuck,' she says, marching over to the weed.

Yes, fucking—that's really what this is all about. Sexual intimacy. Connectedness. Martin might need more time to adjust; he might even need to see a counsellor with her. But she needs to know where they stand, because she isn't done with all that. Not yet.

She pulls out her phone, taps a foot as the extension clicks through. 'Martin, I'm sorry to bother you. I know you said you would be late tonight. You've been great through all this, and I know you need time to catch up on work, focus on yourself for a change. But I really need to talk to you before I see the surgeon tomorrow. I need your input. I can't decide this alone. Can you at least tell me what time you'll be home?' She says it all in one breath.

'I'm sorry, Ann.' There is a different tone from the remoteness of the morning. Shy. Confused. 'I'm trying. I really am. I'd just like things to get back to normal.'

She stares at the dandelion already wilting in her hand. 'I understand—I'd like to get back to normal too,' she says, then ends the call.

~

She pours shiraz into the cut-crystal goblet she no longer saves for parties and holidays. Before preparing dinner, she changed the sheets on her bed to a new Egyptian cotton pair with a high thread count, stuffing the old set in a bag for the second-hand shop.

Through the French doors, a breeze brings the scent of fresh-turned earth from the garden. A romantic spring evening and only nine-thirty. The house is silent. She decides to buy a new clock, one that ticks.

At her desk is an open English–French dictionary. She's spent some time trying to draft a message to Denis: nothing complicated, nothing related to the bigger questions she has, just a simple message of best wishes. She has yet to send it or even to confirm him as a friend.

As she places her wineglass on the shelf above her laptop, her hand slips and knocks a small vase to the floor. It breaks cleanly in two, leaving a little puddle of dingy water and the plant—four bamboo shoots—at her feet. The shoots, each a different height and impossibly green with new growth, remain twisted together at the base. They were a gift from Martin, who said the stems reminded him of their family. She nudges them with her foot. So many roots tangled together.

Denis and Will: both tendrils from her past. She turns to her laptop, finds almost immediately the email address she wants, and types with determination: *Just wondering. In the scheme of things, how important were my breasts to you?* Nothing more. She presses send.

It's a bizarre message, stranger perhaps than the second-hand message from Denis. More a plea to the cosmos than to a real person. She can't picture Will in a complete way, only as the boy in this morning's dream.

He responds with uncanny immediacy: *Wow, Annie. Still not much into foreplay are you? And yes, I'm fine. Thanks for asking.* 😊 *Your breasts? They were lovely. But I was always a leg man, don't you remember? Be well, Will.*

She bangs the laptop shut with a laughing snort. *A leg man.* Right. Who is he trying to kid? But something about the message halts her, and makes her think he suspects what she was really asking. *Be well,* he says.

Breasts, legs, heart. She runs her hands down the front of her shirt, then rests her palm against the left side of her chest. She has what matters. Her breasts may be missing, but they are not what she misses, and she does not need people from her past to tell her what to do.

With Martin, she is well rooted.

A paper towel in hand, she cleans up the puddle on the floor. It takes just a few minutes more to replace the bed linens in the spare room with those from the master suite. The bamboo shoots hold tightly together as she drops them in a vase and places it on the bedside table.

She will wait here in the spare-room bed and, when he arrives, she *will* talk. She will break the habit of avoidance that she and Martin have fallen into over the course of her disease, during months when there was only one subject and one question to answer. But that time is over now, and they must sort through all the other aspects of their lives that have been disarranged. They must establish their new normal.

Glass of wine in hand, she slips between the sheets. The strangeness of the room makes her feel like she is on the cusp of something else. The cotton is smooth, and her heart is real.

The Halo

Ann Calandro

'I don't think I can do this,' I said.

I was flat on my back in a hospital bed, looking up at a doctor and nurse. It was hard to see them clearly without my glasses, which had been smashed to bits. The doctor had just explained to me that he was going to drill four screws into my skull—one on each side of my forehead, above my eyebrows, and one on each side of the back of my skull—and that I needed to be conscious when he did that.

After I spoke, he and the nurse continued to look at me. Neither responded to me.

'Why do I need to be awake?' I asked.

'Because you have to be able to tell us what you are feeling,' the nurse finally said. 'We need to drill far enough so that we can attach the halo firmly, but not too far into your skull.'

I thought about this scenario for a few minutes, as if I had any sort of choice. I had been in an accident a few weeks before, and all the doctors had quickly decided that treating my neck injury without surgery was preferable to operating. I fully agreed with that decision, but I hadn't realized that drilling screws into my skull while I was awake was the next step. So far I had experienced using a bedpan, having my hair washed with dry shampoo, undergoing so many X-rays I was convinced I would soon glow in the dark, and being fed soft foods to minimize my risk of choking while lying down. I was already tired of overcooked fish combined with instant mashed potatoes, and I spent hours each day fantasizing about the crusty breads I would someday eat again. I assumed I would recover fully, since the alternative was too horrible to contemplate.

'And so we need you to lie very still while we drill,' the nurse continued. 'Have you ever done biofeedback?'

'No,' I said. 'I'm pretty sure it won't work for me.' I'd first read about biofeedback in a health magazine: it's a kind of mindfulness that aids in self-regulation of physiological pathways and can lower heart rate, blood pressure, and stress. I had tried meditating once or twice after a bad day at work, but I always ended up thinking about something else.

'Okay, then just hold my hand,' the nurse said. 'You can squeeze it if the pain gets too bad.'

I took her hand. It was warm. Mine was cold. I held hers loosely and politely, as if we had just been introduced at a job interview or other work-related event. The doctor began drilling.

'This isn't too bad!' I said. 'It hurts a little, but I can handle it.'

As soon as those words were out of my mouth, the pain worsened. As soon as the pain worsened, it intensified again. In seconds the pain was terrible.

'This really hurts!' I yelled.

'Hold still!' the doctor shouted back.

'Squeeze my hand!' the nurse commanded.

I squeezed her hand hard, then I squeezed it some more.

'Let's try biofeedback anyway, even if you don't think it will work,' the nurse said. She began describing a beach I was walking along.

'I'm not really a beach person,' I said, or thought I said. 'I burn in the sun. I'm not supposed to be in the sun that much. There's a history of melanoma on both sides of my family. My cousins had all these moles removed.'

But maybe I didn't say any of that, because she kept talking. 'You're walking along the edge of the water. The ocean is so blue. The air is so warm. It's such a beautiful day. The water washes up over your feet and then goes out again. You're walking along the sand, right next to the water. Feel the sun on your shoulders. Feel the water on your feet.'

It did sound beautiful. It sounded like Santa Barbara. I had been to Santa Barbara once, to visit a friend, and we had walked on the beach. I was still gripping the nurse's hand harder than I had ever gripped anyone's hand. I wanted to say, *I'm sorry if I'm hurting you*, but I couldn't speak. All I could do was groan or yell each time I felt the drill, and breathe deeply in the spaces when it stopped. Periodically the doctor would ask me something, and I would answer with a yes or a no.

The nurse kept talking calmly. Being on the beach sounded infinitely preferable to being in the hospital bed, and I began to look frantically for the door that would lead me from where I was to where I wanted to be.

'Just think about being on the beach,' said the nurse. 'You're walking on the beach. You're walking on the beach.'

'I'm walking on the beach,' I repeated, and suddenly I *was* walking on the beach. I was still holding the nurse's hand, but I was no longer squeezing it with my entire being. Her voice was far away. I could feel the salt spray on my face and water on my feet. *I think it worked*, I thought. The pain wasn't as bad as it had been. I could still feel it, but it was muffled as if there were a cotton quilt between the drill and my skull.

'Almost done,' I heard, or thought I heard, the doctor say. Then the sound of the drill stopped.

The nurse took her hand from mine and began flexing her fingers. 'You have some grip' she said, 'but it looked like the biofeedback worked—towards the end, anyway.'

'It finally did,' I said. 'It was the strangest feeling.'

'I can give you some oral pain medication now,' the doctor said. 'The skin around those screws is going to be sore for a little while, but it won't be too bad.'

'Okay,' I said, 'thank you.'

The halo—a padded metal scaffolding around my head connected to a sheepskin-lined molded plastic vest that fit exceptionally tight—was then attached to the screws.

Wearing the halo enabled the bones in my neck and back to heal in the proper position, and one day, several weeks later, I left the hospital, still in the halo, to finish mending at home. Eventually the halo was downgraded to a hard neck brace, then to a soft neck brace, and then to nothing.

Weeks later, I went back to the hospital with thank-you bags of homemade cookies for everyone who had treated me, but I didn't see the nurse who held my hand. No one I asked knew whom I was talking about.

'Could have been an agency nurse, just there for that day,' I was told. 'Could have been someone who left for another job.'

The doctor who had drilled the screws didn't remember her. 'Oh, well,' he said vaguely, running his hand through his thinning hair, 'a lot of nurses work here. I don't know them all.'

~

More than three decades later, I've pretty much gotten back to normal. From time to time I still think of that nurse, though, because I've never succeeded at biofeedback again. But for some years now I've had a recurring dream that reminds me of how it felt.

In this dream, I'm driving down a busy avenue that I know well, and abruptly I'm somewhere else: a small, wonderful neighborhood that I didn't know existed but that I've apparently been dreaming of for years. As soon as I see it, I know it's where I'm meant to be. It's where I need to live. I love everything about it: the people, houses, streets, museums, concert halls, gardens, libraries, schools, restaurants and stores. 'We need to move here right away!' I excitedly tell my husband, who is suddenly next to me in the car. He agrees. We smile at each other in delight. I immediately turn the car around so we can go home and call a realtor and put our house up for sale and begin packing, and then I awaken. I never get past that point in the dream.

'You'd think that just once I could dream I was living in that neighborhood,' I said to my husband the last time this happened, but he was still sleeping.

Although that neighborhood exists only in my dreams, I have been dreaming about it for long enough that it has a place in my memories, too. So it is with biofeedback. I've tried and tried—during an MRI, during childbirth—and it has never worked again, but I have that one memory of it working. I remember the salt air and hot sun on my face and the water on my feet. My hair curled up in the wind. Why did it work that time, and why hasn't it worked since? Was it because of her, that particular nurse? Was it because of me, that particular patient? Was it the combination of the two of us … or something else entirely?

Maybe sometimes, a door does appear in the back wall of the wardrobe, a path unfurls in the forest, and a neighborhood that exists in dreams doesn't vanish when morning comes.

Thicker Than Water

Nicole Zelniker

The main reason Tara Holmes had been caught was that her blood wouldn't clot, and I told her so. Since the victim was her father, she automatically would have been one of the first suspects, but if she hadn't had to call for help after the tussle she might not have been arrested for a while longer.

She seemed to know this—or, at least, she didn't argue when I told her. She came to me twice a week for Advate, which I injected into her veins to stop her from bleeding out.

'Honestly, it's easier to be a hemophiliac in jail,' she told me one day, about a month after her arrival at the prison where I worked in Fargo, North Dakota. 'The other girls pretty much leave me alone. Don't want to be responsible for another life, I think.'

'I certainly wouldn't want to be,' I said, and Tara laughed.

I removed the needle and pressed a cotton ball to her skin. She had been tan when she arrived last month, bruises just barely visible beneath her handcuffs. She had lightened almost to an olive color.

I stuck the bandaid on her skin, and she rolled down her orange sleeve. 'Thanks,' she said. She ran a hand through her dark hair—one of the other girls had cut it up to her shoulder blades—and winked at me. 'See you Tuesday.'

~

Verna had worked at the jail longer than I—nearly twenty years—and I could tell she was a little bitter when I became head nurse. Meghan had more training than I did, but she was pretty fine with it, or that's what she told me at least. 'Besides,' she said, 'the girls all like you best.'

I shrugged. 'Some of them do.' In truth, most of them did, but that was because I didn't pry and tried my best not to judge them. I honestly didn't want to know why these women had been locked up.

I had my own desk in the back and a nameplate on the door in black letters. It was there that the warden told me we were getting a hemophiliac. He came to me every so often with an inmate who needed semi-regular care, but Tara would be the first I'd see every week, twice a week. 'Have you ever dealt with hemophilia before?' he asked.

'No, sir,' I said. 'We learned about it in school, though.'

'She'll need injections,' he said, 'in the veins.'

'Yes, sir.'

'Twice a week.'

'Yes, sir,' I said.

Later, when I got that day's newspaper, I read about Tara, although I didn't realize it was her until the end of the article. A young woman had been arrested after killing her father in the city of Bismarck, about a three-hour drive away. I made the connection when the article mentioned she'd be serving time in Fargo, and that she had called 911 when she wouldn't stop bleeding from a head wound.

~

'Don't you want to know why?' Tara asked me. She was sitting on a cot in the nurse's station after her injection.

'No, ma'am.'

She frowned. 'I would want to know. I'm nosy.'

'I don't want to pry,' I said, putting the used needle in the sharps bin.

She shrugged. 'People like to know what you're in for,' she said. 'I know why all the women on my block are here. But I don't know *why* they did it.' She added, 'My roommate was an arsonist.'

'Oh?'

'She told me,' Tara said. 'I'm curious to know what makes people want to start fires. Aren't you?'

'Not so much,' I said. 'That's not my job.'

Verna walked into the room and glanced over at us on the beds. 'Sorry, ladies, we need the cot. One of the inmates just got shanked.'

Tara stood. 'I'll see you Friday, then,' she said.

'Bye, Tara,' I said.

She left for her cell, Verna staring after her.

'What?' I asked.

Verna turned her eyes to me. 'Nothing,' she said, 'just trying to figure out how she can be so pleasant, and a murderer.'

Before I could say anything back, two guards came in with a young woman, who I would learn had been stabbed by her roommate with a letter opener.

~

A hemophiliac's skin is like a map of their recent life: purple bruising where they banged their shin on the table leg; a greenish smudge from sleeping on their arm funny.

When I saw discoloration on Tara's arm, I asked her what had happened.

She wrinkled her nose. 'I thought you said you didn't pry?' The marks stood out against her paler skin, so blue they were almost black, and red around the edges. They looked new—and in the shape of a handprint.

'It's medical,' I said, rolling up her sleeve further. 'I'm your nurse.'

'Just another inmate,' she said, her hazel eyes not meeting mine.

'Doing what?'

'Jeez, how is *that* medical?'

I swabbed the crook of Tara's arm with antiseptic. 'You're evading,' I said, and plunged the needle into her vein.

'And it's not your business,' she said.

When I'd finished, she held the cotton ball while I placed the sticky plaster over it.

'Thanks,' she mumbled, and left.

My stomach twisted, suggesting I'd done something wrong. Which was silly, since Tara was my patient, not my friend.

~

Later that week, Tara requested to see me for an extra appointment. 'Do you have a minute?'

I put my bag on the desk and nodded, taking a seat.

Tara remained standing. 'It's … um, can they hear us?' she asked, pointing to the nurse's station where Meghan was organizing the afternoon medication and the guard waited.

I pulled the blue paper curtain around the examination bed, creating a thin barrier between us and the rest of the unit. 'Probably not, if we speak quietly.'

Tara took off her shirt to show me bruises like tattoos on her upper arms, lime-green and plum. The handprint on her forearm was still there, fading out to a sickening lemon color.

'Tara—'

'I don't know what to do,' she said, her voice wavering.

'It's not an inmate?' I asked.

'No, a guard. He doesn't make me, you know, just blow him. He says he doesn't want me to bleed out all over him. But he grabs me, and he, you know … I'm still getting him off,' she said with a shaky laugh.

'Are there more?' I asked. I didn't want to know, really, but she pulled up her shirt, and I saw marks on her stomach and side.

'He says if I report him, no one will believe me, even with the handprints,' she said. 'My trial is still a month away.'

I bit my lip. 'I'm sorry. I don't know what to do.'

She sat on one of the cots and put her head in her hands. 'I know. I'm sorry. I just, I needed someone to know, I guess. Which isn't fair to you—'

'Don't say that. I'm glad you told me.' I sat next to her and let her cry. I put my arm around her gently, so as not to press.

~

Weeks passed and Tara still wouldn't tell me his name. But based on the few clues she dropped and her behavior depending on which guard escorted her to my clinic, I narrowed it down to an officer named Brent, who happened to be a close friend of the warden.

I asked Tara if she wanted my help requesting a transfer, but she was waiting for her trial and didn't want to do anything to push it back. 'Besides,' she said, 'no one is going to take care of me like you do.'

'There are nurses at every jail,' I said, but I was secretly touched.

Just three weeks away. Then two weeks. Then one. Tara's trial came quicker than many of the other girls'. Possibly because she was paying for a good lawyer or because she was white, I wasn't sure.

Over the next few days she was shuttled back and forth between the prison and the local courthouse. Once, I was summoned to give her an injection outside the courtroom, but I never went inside. Her stepfather came over to thank me and ask me to sit with the family, but I didn't.

I wasn't at the courthouse when they handed down the verdict. One of the others heard about it before I did. She walked into the nurses' station and said, 'Tara Holmes's decision came back. She's guilty.'

I went to my office and cried.

~

I saw Tara the next day, for one last appointment.

'I'll miss you,' she said.

I gave her a small smile and put the cotton ball on her arm. 'I'll miss you, too.'

Together, we placed the bandaid over the injection site, my gloved fingers on hers. We didn't talk about the trial, or that she was going to be in prison for a long time. I didn't ask for the details. I didn't know if she would want me to.

She stood and said, 'I'll see you Tuesday.'

I laughed. 'See you.'

After Tara left, I read about the rest of her case. The newspapers reported she would be in a prison back in Bismarck. At the time of her arrest, her lawyer had told reporters that her father had abused her and her brother. When she'd found out her father was going to become the stepfather to a little girl, she asked him to meet with her.

Before she shot him, he came at her with a knife, threatening her as he demanded she stay away from his new family. She'd only just turned eighteen the month before she arrived at Fargo.

When I handed in my resignation to the warden, he stared at the paper in his hand as if it were written in code. 'I don't understand,' he said. 'I gave you a promotion.'

'I know, sir. And thank you for that.'

He gaped at me as I left. I hoped Verna would become head nurse, because if she got passed over again, she just might quit, too.

~

I didn't mind the long drive to Bismarck—I had time now that I was unemployed and all. The prison was sort of like the jail in Fargo but bigger. Several women in orange jumpsuits were out in the yard. I sat in my car for a while before going in, even though I knew the visiting time was ticking away. Was this fair to Tara? Would she even want to see me?

Eventually, I went inside. The metal detectors and security guards were just like at Fargo. The guards took me to a large room with long tables and told me to wait. There were two other visitors, each talking to a different woman.

After a minute, a guard brought Tara inside. Her eyes widened, and her face split into a grin. She would have got in trouble for running, but she walked as quickly as she could and pulled me into a hug. 'You even came on a Friday,' she said. The guard tapped her shoulder, and she stepped away, taking a seat across the table. 'How did you get here?'

'I drove,' I said.

'Three hours?'

'Well, I'm, uh, I took the day off.'

Tara laughed. The bruise at the corner of her mouth was still there, but faded. It was greenish-brown now, healing.

The Old Doctor and His Waiting Room

C.A. Rivera

The old doctor, buoyed by the energy of the morning crowd rushing the train platform, pulled himself up from the wooden bench, adjusted his gray fedora and waited for the speeding train to come to a stop. For a brief instant, he felt like the screeching subway cars: necessary and frail. On the train he sat near the center door as he always did, opened his newspaper and began reading the horoscopes.

The old doctor, one of the few from his generation still practicing, belonged to a different time. He was trapped between World War II and September 11—this was his history, although he didn't want it to be.

Trembling, he flicked through the newspaper. Unable to recall where he was heading, he closed his eyes and tried to ignore the gnawing he felt in his midgut. He blinked his eyes and yawned, overcome by unrelenting fatigue.

The old doctor got off the train at the last stop, where an elevator took him up to the street level. He paced back and forth in the rain, crossed the street, then crossed back. He sought shelter underneath the awning of a corner store, cleared his throat and tried to remember where he was heading. He had a hunch his clinic was nearby but, unsure in which direction to walk, he hailed a cab.

'Pizza parlor over there,' the old doctor said to the driver.

'Sir, where is over there?'

'Over there, in front of the pizza parlor.'

'Sir, which pizza parlor? There are a thousand pizza parlors.'

'The one in front of my clinic—the old clinic.'

'Old clinic? The pizza parlor in front of your old clinic? I need more information, sir.'

'The pizza parlor in front of my clinic.'

'Sir?'

'I mean the pizza parlor next to the dollar store.'

'What's the clinic address? What are the cross streets? Sir, do you have a card or anything with your address on it?'

'Address?'

'Yeah, address.'

'Let me check.' Rustling, then silence.

'Sir, did you check?'

'Check what?'

'Do you have a letter or card with your address?'

'I don't know.'

'Do you have anything in your pocket with your clinic address, sir? Or in your wallet?'

'Wallet! Yes, I have my wallet. What did you want again?'

'May I have one of those cards there, sir?'

'Yes.' The old doctor's head was throbbing, and he could barely summon the energy to remove his wet green cardigan. He couldn't remember why he was heading to the clinic.

'This must be it. We're here, Doctor.'

'Excuse me?'

'We are here, Doc. That'll be $13.50.'

'Here?' the old doctor asked. 'Where?'

'The corner clinic, across the street from the pizza parlor and next to the dollar store.'

'It's raining.'

'No worries, I'll pull up closer.'

'Okay, thanks. Here's ten dollars, keep the change.'

'Ten dollars, what change?' muttered the driver as the old doctor closed the cab door.

~

The clinic was on the first floor; the waiting room was small. On the door to the back rooms, the word 'doctor' was painted in several languages: Doctor, Medico, Lekarza. Across from the receptionist window hung a reproduction of *Café Terrace at Nigh*t by Vincent van Gogh, and in the center of the back wall was a dusty picture of a boat at sea.

The old doctor walked through the waiting room, back to his office. His nurse, Teresa, greeted him before letting out a deep breath as she flipped the old wooden sign to 'open'. The clinic's volume had decreased over the past year, after his staff had told him to reduce his hours over the previous two years. His entire medical team had left and obtained other jobs, except for Teresa.

This morning she was preparing the three clinic rooms for consultations when an immigrant mother and her young daughter entered the waiting room. The girl was cupping her right ear and moaning. Her mother sat down to fill out the intake paperwork.

Meanwhile, Teresa rushed to answer the phone. 'Do you want me to call an ambulance, Ms Blumenthal?' she asked the caller. 'Please try and come in, if you can.'

As the old doctor headed into his office, he wished he had time to sneak in a quick nap. But before he could sit down, Teresa was knocking on his door, telling him that the girl and her mother were in Room Three.

'Which direction is Room Three again?' he mumbled to himself.

The girl was squirming on the examination table, chewing on the tips of her braids to help soothe the pain. The old doctor sat on his stool, pulled an index card from his white coat pocket and began asking the mother questions. He shared a story about his last trip to Oaxaca, as the family was from there.

Before he could finish, the girl screamed and leaped off the exam table, startling him. 'It hurts!' she yelled. 'My ear hurts!'

'Okay, okay, let's calm down. Can you sit, please?' He grabbed the otoscope to look in her ear. 'Oh, that's infected.'

'Ouch! Make it go away, Doctor.'

'Away we will make it go. Ear infections often go away on their own, but this one has been there for some time, so I need to give you medication.'

'Infection?' asked the mother. 'Medication?'

'I'll write the prescription,' said the old doctor to the girl and her mother as he walked out of the room and towards his office.

A few moments later Teresa knocked on his door, waking him. 'The mother is asking for the prescription. Have you written it yet?'

The nurse shuffled through papers on his desk. 'The mother also said you didn't answer her questions.'

'Prescription? Questions?'

'Yes, for the girl's ear infection.'

'Oh, yes, the infection … Where was the infection again?'

'In the ear, Doctor. I'll wait here so I can give the prescription to them. Also, Ms Blumenthal is in Room One, and two other patients are in the waiting room.'

Teresa snatched the prescription from his hand. After she gave it to the mother, she guided her and the girl to the door of the clinic. 'This is our last day,' Teresa told them. 'The clinic is closing for good, take care.' She went to the break room to get some coffee and found the old doctor looking for his mug.

'Have you seen Ms Blumenthal yet?' asked Teresa from the doorway.

'Ms Blumenthal?' asked the old doctor.

'Yes, Ms Blumenthal—she is in Room One. She's in severe back pain, screaming.'

'Screaming?' The old doctor tipped his head to the side, listening. 'What room?'

'Room One, Doctor. I'll find your cup and bring a coffee to you.'

He walked out of the break room, thinking about the warm coffee that would soon be brought to him, and headed to his office. He sat at his desk and began to read his newspaper; soon he was dozing.

Teresa barged in. 'Doctor?'

'Yes?'

'Ms Blumenthal is still in Room One.'

'Room One?'

Teresa escorted the old doctor to Room One, where Ms Blumenthal was wincing and holding her back.

'No chocolates today?' the old doctor asked her.

'Chocolates?' she said. 'I can barely move.' She tried to straighten and look at him, groaning in the process.

He turned pale. 'We need to call an ambulance.'

'Please do!' cried Ms Blumenthal.

'Teresa, call the 911 dispatcher,' yelled the old doctor to his nurse, who nodded. 'They'll be here soon, so try to hang on, Ms Blumenthal. Take some deep breaths.'

He hurried to his office and sat at his desk, his heart thumping. He wrapped his clammy hands around the coffee mug, dipped the tip of his nose into the steam and closed his eyes. He tried to remember how he knew Ms Blumenthal. He thought maybe she lived upstairs.

~

After arranging the ambulance, Teresa called in the other two patients. In Room Two she placed Yakubu, the neighborhood hobo who spoke limited English and only talked to people he knew in Harlem. He could hear Ms Blumenthal moaning in agony through the wall as he sat at the edge of the exam table, his fingertips pressing against his abdomen. He was thin with pasty black skin and deep sunken eyes. He suffered from constipation and came to the clinic once a month for a mineral oil enema. Teresa told him she would return shortly, then left to place the last patient in Room Three.

Cisco was a thin, tall man who wore dark shades and walked with a limp. He'd lost fifty pounds in the past six months while undergoing chemotherapy for urinary tract cancer. He despised going to the hospital, so he came to the clinic to get his Foley catheter exchanged. Teresa informed him she'd be back as soon as she could.

When she returned to her desk, she rested her head in her hands and wondered if she should tell the patients this was the last time the old doctor would see them. The sign on the front door advised that the clinic would be closing soon, but she was unsure if the patients had seen or read the sign.

She walked into the break room, sat on a chair and sobbed. She couldn't hold it in any longer. As the only nurse left, she did almost everything, from checking in patients to billing, as well as tasks she had inherited while working with the old doctor. She wiped her eyes, swollen from crying, their lids thick and stuck together.

A banging on the clinic's front door brought her back to the present. She wiped her eyes and went to let the emergency personnel in. Cisco and Yakubu watched the medical technicians as they entered Room One. They carefully strapped Ms Blumenthal to their stretcher and wheeled her out, en route to the hospital ER.

Teresa administered the mineral oil enema to Yakubu and left him making loud noises on the toilet. She exchanged Cisco's Foley catheter, then saw both patients out rather swiftly.

'I'm done,' she said to the empty room. She headed over to tap on the old doctor's door. 'Doctor? Can I come in?' There was no response, so she slowly walked into his office. 'Doctor?'

'I was just resting my eyes. Preparing for the long day.'

'I think the day is over.'

'It went quick.'

'Do you want me to help you close up?'

'Oh no, I'll be here late. Preparing for next week.'

Teresa went out to the waiting room. Her hair and mascara were a mess. She would settle the last of the accounts over the next two weeks. But she was still unclear about how exactly things would end.

As she left, she flipped the sign to 'Closed' and locked the door behind her.

~

The old doctor looked at the charts piled up on his desk. He couldn't recall which patients he'd seen today. He walked into the quiet waiting room. He sat on a chair and stared at the receptionist window, trying to remember what it was he had gone out there for.

He glanced outside. He was hungry. He headed across the street to Lou's pizza parlor.

'Hey, Doc, you want the usual?'

'Where's the boss?'

'In the back, getting the dough ready for tomorrow.'

'So, the boss is counting the dough?'

'Good one, Doc. A large slice, and an orange can—eat in or takeout?'

'Put it in a paper bag for me.'

'Do you need a ride home, Doc? Lou's just about done, and I know he'd be happy to take you.'

But the old doctor did not remember where he lived; he only recognized specific landmarks such as the burger stand by his home. As he politely turned down the ride, he was scared and eager to go back to his clinic. It was getting dark as he walked unsteadily across the road in the rain. He would catch a cab home later.

The old doctor sat facing the reproduction Van Gogh in the waiting room. He picked up his slice of pizza and let the tip bend into his mouth, savoring the oily cheese he loved. He stared at the painting for a long time as he tried to remember why it was special to him. Then he recalled that he and his wife had been painted into an artist's version of *Café Terrace at Night.* The old doctor had commissioned the artist to paint them sitting at one of the tables with a bottle of wine in the center, toasting each other.

He finished his slice of pizza, drank his orange soda and belched a few times. As he continued to admire the painting, he could not hold back tears when he remembered giving it to his wife.

The old doctor lay down on the row of chairs, still mesmerized by the picture. After a while he rolled onto his back, stared at the ceiling, closed his eyes and remembered listening to his wife read the obituaries of famous people over dinner. His mouth sagged open, and he fell asleep.

The sensor light turned off. In the darkness of the waiting room, the old doctor found refuge. His snores echoed throughout the room, drowning out the rain, and lightning flickered in through the large window that was glazed with fog.

You Brachy, You Buyee

Scott Dalgarno

Few things have gotten my attention like these words: 'Dr T— brought your case up at the Tumor Board this morning.'

I received this message from Bob, my Radiation Oncologist's physician's assistant, having gone in to hear the results of a PET scan I'd had the week before.

'Good news!' said the PA. 'Your cancer is localized. It's not in your bones. We're hopeful it's still curable.'

'Thank you so much, Bob,' are *not* the words that came out of my mouth. I was familiar with him: a personable fellow, and very professional. We'd spent the first five minutes talking about the yard sale he and his wife were putting on that coming weekend.

But Bob tended to alarmism. This I knew.

A year before, when my prostate-specific antigen (PSA) had gone up from near-zero to near-zero plus zero-point-one, he'd asked if I was having any bone pain. *Bone pain?* A quick Google led me to see that a person with a PSA as low as mine who has had brachytherapy for prostate cancer—as I'd had five years before—shouldn't be suffering from anything more serious than the pain associated with a regular blood draw to check levels. 'No,' I'd said quickly.

A year later, the PSA had risen a bit higher, and Dr T— had ordered the PET.

I'd found the scan itself to be easy, just twenty minutes scooting backward and forward like an auto mechanic while the tech made sure to check all the bones and organs between my neck and knees. Dressing after, I couldn't read him at all. I had no idea if he'd found a mass the size of a grapefruit somewhere, or if I was in the clear.

Now, Bob had just told me that my tumor was small and isolated in one quadrant of my prostate. My pelvis looked normal, and there was no sign of any lymph node involvement. That was the extent of his good news.

The Tumor Board, Bob explained, was a collection of urologists, radiological oncologists, and other physicians and assistants who had met that morning. I imagined a roomful of major players looking at my pelvis blown up a hundred times its size on a screen that hung from a huge wall. It sounded a little like one of Sarah Palin's 'death panels'.

'The Tumor Board—' Did Bob have to use the T-word so many times? '—are in agreement that you need to have your bladder scoped. The neck—' *My bladder has a neck?* '—is thickened, and they are suspicious about that. You will, of course, also need a biopsy of your prostate. The urologists handle those procedures. That's their area.'

'That's their area' was key here, as I would shortly learn. Like any other institution, cancer hospitals have turf wars, and I'd become a brand-new pawn. But how expendable was I going to be, and to whom?

My brachytherapist signed off on the Tumor Board's plan, but I had no idea if he was really enthusiastic about it or merely agreeable because that's how things work in such places. I pictured him bowing like a Zen monk to the Department of Urology whenever brachytherapy *failure* was suspected.

Bob had suggested I might need to have 'salvage surgery' and volunteered that such surgery was messy, at best. Brachytherapy effectively cooks the prostate, and what's left is not unlike meat you have to scrape out of a pan after roasting. I'd known this going into it, six years before, but I was also acquainted with the fact that such therapy not only kills cancer cells within the prostate but also has a halo effect, meaning that it kills any renegade cancer cells that might have escaped the organ by a few centimeters. This fact sold me.

Okay, I also liked the thought of not being filleted.

~

Two weeks after speaking with Bob, I was in the office of a young urologist, Dr L—, whose services I had politely refused six years before when, after consultation with him, I'd chosen a radiological approach. Might this be an I-told-you-so moment? *Mr Dalgarno, I see you have come crawling back to this office, dragging your roasted prostate between your …* If he was thinking that, there was no sign, although he surely thought I had made a huge mistake by forgoing surgery and choosing a Mickey Mouse alternative. I imagined him smirking and saying, 'You brachy, you buyee'—the Pottery Barn theory of prostate radiation therapy.

He seemed too circumspect to say anything like that, but whereas Bob had said that my tumor was small and isolated, Dr L— disagreed. He said that my whole prostate 'lit up' (a term my daughter uses to describe killing bad guys in her favorite video game) on the scan. My bladder was lit as well.

This was clearly serious. 'We will likely be taking out the prostate and a number of lymph nodes,' Dr L— said.

He was very professional, if a little too eager to clean up my previous therapist's massive 'failure'. But I was pleased to hear he could scope my bladder then and there. *Scope now, scrape later*, I thought. The idea of having to give up my bladder and wear a bag on my leg and smell forever like a nursing home was definitely preying on me. I needed to know how bad this was going to be, and quickly.

'Have you had a catheter inserted before?' he asked.

'Yes, but that was under anesthesia when I had my procedure.'

'Oh,' he said, apologetically.

This time there was genuinely good news: the screen showing the video captured by the tiny camera that was touring my privates was in view. Even my unschooled eyes could see there was nothing suspicious, just healthy tissue. The inside of my bladder was a lovely duckling yellow that reflected the light. Narrow blood vessels lined it, revealing the shape of a balloon.

'A healthy bladder,' he acknowledged, 'for a man your age.'

'Good to know,' I said. I was too ecstatic to quibble about my age. No bladder bag would be needed. Yes! Everything checked out, including the quadrant of the prostate visible as the scope was—ouch!—pulled out.

'Once you have the biopsy,' he said, 'we'll have you come in to discuss next steps.'

My enthusiasm dampened as quickly as it had risen.

~

Bob had given me hope that the biopsy would be mercifully short and MRI guided. And if only one quadrant of the prostate was suspicious, why sample the whole thing?

No such luck. The biopsy would involve a shotgun approach, and a prolonged shotgunning at that.

Six years before, I'd had twelve core samples drawn with as many needles, confirming the original diagnosis of cancer; this time, sixteen samples would be drawn. Between biopsies I'd forgotten how that procedure felt. Thankfully, physical pain is somewhat forgettable.

As I lay there in a fetal position, Dr L—'s assistant began my slow torture. In the next moment I had remembered the sound of the 'gun' they use and, with it, the dull pain with each shot into my organ. The prostate may have been rendered retrograde by brachytherapy, but damn it hurt, and every time.

She told me to expect blood, 'lots of blood', the first couple of times I urinated. And blood upon ejaculation too. She looked at me with questioning eyes. I tried to appear as opaque as possible.

~

A week later I got the word: a simple phone call from another of the urologist's staff. 'No cancer,' he said.

Really? I thought. *No cancer?* After the word 'tumor' had been thrown around as often as the word 'margarita' on Cinco de Mayo? And after so much of me had 'lit up' like a Christmas tree?

'We did find some benign tissue in one or two of the cores,' he said.

Benign. I knew that was a good word.

It took me a few seconds to realize that my prostate was growing back, six years after my radiation therapy. Back then, my brachytherapist had said he believed the procedure had rendered it a ball of jelly, a globe of dead tissue that would just sit there until the rest of me died. But that was clearly not the case; my prostate was making a comeback. The biopsy and the climbing PSA numbers confirmed this.

'There's no need for you to come in and see anyone,' said the urologist's PA, adding, 'Funny thing, the prostate gland.'

Yeah, I thought, *I can live with that.*

Win a Date with John Mayer!

D.E.L.

As a teen, my all-time favorite movie was *Win a Date with Tad Hamilton!* It stars Kate Bosworth as Rosalee, a blonde farmgirl who wins a once-in-a-lifetime date with Tad Hamilton (Josh Duhamel). Rosalee and Tad try to fall in love, but ultimately their relationship goes down in flames. Ever since the film's release in 2004, my world has revolved around the scenario of winning a date with a celebrity and fantasizing a happier ending for myself.

There was a time where I would recite memorized lines to the point that my best friend, Elle, would roll her eyes in annoyance. We would banter during late-night sleepovers in the seventh grade about which celebrity our Win a Date scenario would be with. Chewing gobs of Extra Classic Bubble Gum to practice making out with our delectable victims of passion while we watched *Win a Date*, we would speak endlessly of our unrequited love for certain famous men we could only dream of dating.

This leads me to my next obsession: John Mayer.

I can't help being hopelessly devoted to the world-famous star who now hosts the Instagram talk show *Current Mood.* I even owned a leather satchel with his face plastered on both sides, a bespoke creation purchased as a winning bid on eBay back in 2004 as a present for my thirteenth birthday. This was in addition to the fourth-row tickets to see John Mayer himself at an amphitheatre in Chula Vista, featuring Maroon 5 as the warm-up act. I went rocking my new accessory.

In our first three years of high school, my close friends and I celebrated John's birthday. Each year I held my nifty purse in my lap while we sang 'Happy Birthday', then I made a wish on behalf of my imaginary lover and devoured a cookie in his honor.

I became with child at the tender age of sixteen, and thus

attended California State University, Bakersfield, during what would have been my senior year.

~

I'm not completely to blame for falling so madly for John Mayer. The guitar hero is dashing. His looks are superior. He has a perfect sense of humor. He succeeded in the online Bottle Cap Challenge, that recently went viral.

'And my, what big hands you have!' I imagine saying to him.

He might respond, 'All the better to play this six-string damsel, or to hold you in the midst of existential distress, my dear.'

But as I age into my thirties, I can't help but need to confide in someone that I am twenty-eight and my *Win a Date with John Mayer!* plan hasn't come to fruition.

I still have the sublime confidence that if he waltzed into the room—preferably the customer entrance of my pop's screen-printing warehouse in Bakersfield—John could be the Tad Hamilton and I the Rosalee; it would be love at first sight of my light-blue eyes.

I would've liked to show him the bag, but it was either lost in a recent move or at one of his shows in the 2017 California Mid-State Fair, kinda like Cinderella's glass slipper.

~

Let's delve more into my experiences with this purse, because I sported that sucker around for years with great pride and enthusiasm, as though it was a public display of affection.

Visualize a condensed vinyl album—or two, in fact, because the bag was square. Gracing each surface was John on the front cover of a magazine. One was an early 2000s *Guitar Player* issue headlined 'The Blues Lust & Ferocious Chops of an Unabashed Pop Star'. The other, an *Acoustic* issue, showed the beyond-gorgeous squire in very casual attire: a navy zip-up hoodie and a white tee. His bed-headed smirk was sublime.

The bag possessed a certain energy, permitting the individual who properly functioned with it to radiate a striking aura along with a certain *je ne sais quoi*. I would switch the sides of the bag around depending on my mood. The *Acoustic* cover was meant for hotboxing sessions with my friends, as John was noticeably more relaxed, while the *Guitar Player* cover helped to convey my goddess-like prowess. And imagine the compliments I received!

I *always* had the bag in hand. We walked *together*, hand in pouch and arm in strap; my friends referred to me and the bag as *us* and *them*. At my volleyball tournaments in Los Angeles, where I got to flaunt my assets in tight spandex, John was *always* there to hold my belongings and motivate me to kick ass. At guitar lessons he would keep my picks in that stellar leather pocket and just totally be the light of inspiration to riff along like I was the star of the show. We were a fantasy couple.

By the time I turned fourteen, I was *married* to that bag. Married. *Mayer-ried*. As well as my things, it carried his albums and an iPod filled to the brim with bootleg recordings of his unreleased songs.

But, in all reality, this was my fantasy that I chose to live in. *This is my bubbly personality*, as my Facebook tagline once read. *Bottled blonde, bottled champagne, bottled emotions. Pop the champagne, I am bubbly.*

But this isn't just a story about a lady with a personality disorder who hoards crap in a crappy bag, and I mean that with great compassion.

~

In the heat of summer 2013, I was misusing the psychotropic medications prescribed to me after my provisional diagnosis of bipolar disorder. Meanwhile, John was on tour and had a show at the California Mid-State Fair on July twenty-second, just over a week after my birthday, July thirteenth.

I remember what happened like it was yesterday.

My father generously spared me some cash, so I decided to get a much-needed mani-pedi at a spa downtown near his warehouse. I had my driver's license, and the Volkswagen Passat lemon of a car happened to be functioning, which was a very rare occasion. I was counting down the days to see John Mayer play where I had once seen Britney Spears frolic to '… Baby One More Time'.

While on my makeover expedition I had the husband satchel in hand and was doing particularly fine until I left the salon and ventured to the Starbucks across the street, where I ordered an unsweetened iced green tea. Upon receiving my drink, I noticed that the straws weren't green but an unbearable and ungodly *red*, as the store had completely run out of their trademark *green straws*.

For some reason, this triggered my mental state into *psychosis*. I went from curiosity about the red straw, to staring at John's face on the bag, to looking at my fresh long pearlescent nails, to staring at my ring finger, to staring at John's face again—then eventually I assumed that *I really was married to John Mayer*.

As this continued, I somehow wandered down yonder to my friend Cam's house and spent the night, while my delusions only became more enhanced. It was just a coincidence that John Mayer, aka *the* love of my life, was performing on my birthday at the Central Coast where I grew up, but I thought he doing this solely for *me*. This belief had sparked an abundance of emotions that I had no idea what to do with. I was rather elated, my sheer mania blending with my unique sense of serendipity.

'Cam!!! I *have* to get to Paso Robles—my husband will be there! *Believe me, I AM MARRIED to the man on my purse!*' I kept desperately trying to explain this to her, over and over again. 'My car is starting to break down already. And, ya know something? My parents won't even let me take the damn thing. Let's book the Amtrack.'

Cam finally gave me her two cents, saying, 'If you get your ass to the train, I will give you everything I have just so you make it to Paso. I'll pay for your fair ticket, too, but your husband's got you for admission to the show and whatever happens after.'

After I awoke from a deep sleep, I received a phone call from my mama explaining that she was going to send me to visit my best friend in Hawaii for a week. Although it wasn't obvious to me at the time, I've since realised that my family had tired of my delusional thoughts and musings. That year alone, I had been admitted to the Good Samaritan psychiatric hospital twice in only a few months. My sound belief that I was wife to the artist had hit a sour note with my family. To be honest, I was kicked out of my house that night because

I was in a frenzy over attending the concert, *plus* I had gotten two stellar John Mayer tattoos that day.

At this point in my medical misdiagnosis rollercoaster 'round the depths of hell, I believed I was just a naturally quirky girl and *nothing was wrong*, so I refused to take my medication. I would delightfully throw the pills on the bathroom carpet as if watering them twice daily would grow them into pretty daisies.

I had paid for the tattoos with a nifty bag of quarters—$75 worth, to be exact—at a parlor downtown. After having the hopeful epiphany that I should live in the moment for the sake of love, I arrived at the parlor knowing exactly what I wanted. I showed the tattoo artist a graphic of a broken heart logo from Google that was tagged as 'Heartbreak Warfare', a Mayer song. The artist tattooed a blue broken heart on my right wrist and *Johnny* on my right upper thigh in red pirate-style script. Classy, right?

Needless to say, I missed John's Mid-State Fair appearance in 2013. I did, however, spend the night cradling my satchel in bed at my friend's home as if I were snuggling with the man of my dreams.

When I look back on that time, what hits me the hardest is my innocent fantasy of just wanting to be held, just wanting to be loved, by a man worthy of my dreams. There's a purity and safety in that kind of love that I longed for later in young adulthood when relationships often left me in deep despair.

~

Can these experiences be seen as valid reasons for why I should win the date with John Mayer? Just how charming is a woman's insanity? I'm reminded of the It's Happy Bunny phrase popular in 2003 when I was muddling through junior high: 'cute but psycho'.

Don't worry, everything is fine today. No one is getting married—I am faithful to my god-sent therapist.

To wrap up this cute but psycho love story that I know I will never move on from—I mean, these tattoos just won't wash off—it should be noted that I was admitted into the UCLA Resnick Neuropsychiatric Hospital shortly after this psychotic episode. I had spent two long months trying to pretend everything was fine, in order to avoid having to face another hospitalization. But after my admission, I trotted around the facility with the new ink on my wonderland, realizing that it was a reason and a way to celebrate my life.

I have never been in love, and I have been deeply hurt by the men who have interrupted my life, but I have the feeling of a love song tattooed on my wrist. I can't worry about all these emotions and experiences that I have yet to get in touch with—*I shouldn't.* I have my amazing daughter, who is full of the only love I need, and we're busy conquering the world as a dynamic duo.

So, my tattoos have a *very* significant and sincere meaning to me. A semicolon tattoo is a symbol for suicide awareness and recovery, and my John Mayer tattoos are a symbol of the strength, love, pride and dignity that I feel when I listen to his music. That *is* love when I am in the midst of all that mania. Because I can't help but think it could be an adorable thing, to be so crazy it tugs at your heartstrings.

Doctor's Appointment

Rebecca Garnett Haris

Sophie's thighs spill over the sides of the plastic National Health Service chair. Her foot taps up and down. She chews her nails then wraps her arms under her pendulous stomach, a consequence of years of eating junk food; she stashes crisps and Coca-Cola under the bed, a secret eater. She stares out of the window, grass-green eyes blank. Different from my other two children, she views the world in a tapestry stitched with greys instead of pinks, greens and blues. I first noticed it when she didn't reach for toys at the mother-and-toddler group and rode her trike around the circle of children playing at a Christmas party, oblivious to the delights of others as Santa showered them with gifts.

Red hair splays over her hunched shoulders; unwashed, matted and with split ends, it hasn't felt the scratch of a brush for a month. The cheap body spray we bought in Superdrug last week was her choice—she insisted it had to be that brand. It wafts into the GP's waiting room every time she moves, but underneath I can still sense a mouldy smell.

~

'A special offer,' the shop assistant said, holding up the can, turning her back on her smirking colleague. She leant closer to me as I paid the bill. 'My cousin Anthea reminds me of your friend.'

Sophie stood at the edge of the door, hands in her pockets. I was relieved she couldn't hear, as my heart sank at the young woman's attempt to ingratiate me into her disability club.

She kept talking. 'And God knows how difficult that was. My auntie phoning my mum in the night, coming to ours every day, crying at the kitchen table as Mum patted her on the back and gave her loads of tea.' She tore off the receipt. 'How old is she, your friend?'

‘She’s my daughter,’ I said, folding the receipt into my purse.

‘Never. You don’t look old enough.’

I smiled at her and swallowed my irritation. She was just trying to be kind.

Sophie pulled on my arm as we walked through the shopping centre. ‘Told you that brand. Saw it online. It was going cheap.’

‘Okay, that’s the brand, then.’

My pulse quickened because I knew what was about to happen. For the next hour, my daughter obsessed over the fact that I had wanted to buy another brand. On and on she repeated the same words.

~

Sophie’s hand, damp and limp, sits in my palm. I watch other patients read their magazines and type their messages and scroll down their phones, but the quick glances and whispering make my shoulders tense.

They see an obese, unkempt red-haired girl. She’s in her lumberjack outfit, as my older daughter calls it: a man’s oversize plaid shirt, men’s baggy black jeans and her sand-coloured hiking boots. They don’t see her quick mind that memorises recipes, telephone numbers and map details. They don’t see her lack of guile and vitriol.

Her eyes are tender but fearful as they scan the room, a cacophony clanging in her brain.

~

She told me on Sunday afternoon, a week before her GP appointment. It was marked on the calendar, *Sophie to see Dr Croft*, in big red letters with a smiley next to them. I’d shown it to her every day that week; she’d stared at it with blank eyes, saying nothing, just flicking her fingers and humming to herself.

That Sunday, she blurted something out in a loud monotone, and Liam turned up the TV. I glared at him and mouthed, ‘Pause it.’ He shook his head, threw the remote on the sofa and walked out of the room. I picked up the remote and pressed pause.

'My hands get wet,' Sophie shouted. 'There's a drum in my head, and I can't breathe!' She looked at peeling wallpaper in the corner of our sitting room. Her head moved from side to side.

'Sophie, look at me.' I sat on the edge of the sofa and touched her arm.

She flinched. 'Can't do it, Mum.'

~

But she has done it, and we are here in the waiting room. I cough to clear the lump forming in my throat as I squeeze her hand. She pulls it away.

A young man, my son's age, comes to the door of the waiting room and calls her name. He's whippet-thin with eager eyes gleaming through horn-rimmed glasses, ready to put into practice the latest NICE—National Institute for Health and Care Excellence—guidelines. Without a stitch of clothing out of place, he's all neatly contained lines right down to his shiny brogues.

My heart sinks, and I prepare for the mantras: *You need to lose weight. Are you eating your five fruit and veg a day*? Or the corker for someone like Sophie, who would rather sit in a darkened room day after day than try to integrate with a group of people: *Have you tried a group Weight Watchers class*?

This encounter, it seems, will be like another humiliating meeting with a young person not much older than my autistic daughter.

~

Two years ago, I attended a parents' evening at Sophie's school. An occasion that's uplifting and encouraging if your child is a Grade A student, belongs to the debate club and is responsible for the winning goal in the end-of-year netball tournament—not so good if your child 'isn't giving her best' or 'finds it difficult to interact with peers'.

'Mrs Harmon, we're concerned about Sophie.' The teenage-looking teacher leant forward across the desk from me. *Why are these teachers and doctors SO young?*

There was pity in her eyes, and the familiar flip in my stomach. I scrabbled in my handbag for a tissue. 'Sorry, bit of a cold.' I blew my nose hard, hoping the noise and the movement would re-centre me so I wouldn't start sobbing in a full room. As I glanced around, I noticed most parents had their daughters with them. Mine had refused to come. Not surprising—at least she was consistent.

'Sorry, what were you saying?' I asked, looking straight at her teacher.

'We're just concerned about Sophie in her break times.'

'I thought she was doing fine during her breaks? I know she's not the most sociable, but when I ask if she talks to the other girls she always says yes.'

'Sophie sits in the toilet for a lot of break times. When someone else needs the cubicle she refuses to come out, and it's causing distress to the other girls. She also stands by herself in the corner of the cafeteria spinning in circles.'

The disappointment started in the pit of my stomach and worked its way up into my throat where it sat, constricting my words. 'Really? She told me she's made friends and chats to Laura a lot?'

'I'm afraid not,' the teacher said, breaking eye contact and opening a folder, seemingly embarrassed by my daughter's lying.

I sat, momentarily grieving the loss of Laura.

'I think we need some strategies … ' the teacher began.

I stood suddenly, saliva filling my mouth. 'I need to go. I'll be in touch.'

In the car, I cried.

We created a strategy, Sophie's teacher and I, once my disappointment had settled. Sophie was given a lunchtime buddy.

But Sophie's constant circling of the buddy led her to complain to her parents that dizziness was affecting her schoolwork.

After all the strategies failed, I started home-schooling Sophie. No more parents' evenings, or barricading in the toilets, or spinning in the cafeteria. Sophie just sat in her bedroom staring at the computer screen, chewing paper and occasionally laughing at cat videos on YouTube. I begged her to engage with some textbooks and final exam practice papers.

~

'Sophie Harmon?' The doctor's voice breaks through my thoughts.

The flicking. Thumb and third finger. Don't know why third. Both hands.

Sophie is staring at the GP, and tiny beads of sweat are forming at her hairline. The look of terror in her eyes has a life of its own.

I press my hand into her lower back. 'Count to ten slowly, Sophie. You can do it.' I'm aware of people looking at us: teenagers giggling; pensioners muttering, *I blame it on the parents;* a businessman straightening his tie, crossing and uncrossing his legs as he hides behind his newspaper.

The doctor's office reeks of family and positivity and success. Photographs of laughing groups of children, award ceremonies and sports days clutter his desk. Above it is a photo of his perfect family in their skiing gear, standing on a white mountain somewhere: a beaming wife with perfect bone structure, the boy's head thrown back in laughter, and the girl snuggled into her father, flecks of snow settling on her cheeks.

This is what autism has done to me. Jealousy holds me in its green jaws as I gaze at the peace and calmness of others' lives. My fight just to be okay is relentless, and the guilt of wanting to live like them erodes me.

The doctor tells us to sit, motioning for my daughter to be next to him. He's arranged the chairs so we are facing him in a semicircle. He leans towards my daughter. 'Hello, Sophie, I'm Doctor Croft. It's nice to meet you.' His eyes are kind and soft as he talks to my daughter.

Head down, she mumbles behind the curtain of her hair.

'Doctor, we're here today …' I start.

He puts his finger to his lips then points to my daughter. She can't see this movement as she hides behind her tangled hair. The irritation sits in my throat, and I curb the anger behind my breastbone.

'A little bird tells me you like Marvel films?' he says and smiles at Sophie.

The curtain of hair sways, and she lifts her head, bewilderment in her eyes. 'A little bird told you?' She looks around the room. 'Where is it? Birds speak?'

Dr Croft shakes his head, grimaces and looks at me as if to say 'what a twat'. I mentally agree but say nothing for fear of starting a scene and walking out. That parents' evening taught me a lesson: issues will still need to be resolved even if I walk away from them.

And I'm intrigued that he knows about Sophie's obsession with Marvel. How did he find that out?

'No, sorry, Sophie,' he says. 'There are no birds in here. It's just a saying.'

A saying my daughter has taken literally. I'm surprised she hasn't bolted out of the room after imagining talking birds.

He starts again, attempting to redeem himself. 'Which character in Marvel do you like best, Sophie?'

I can see her grinning behind her hair. 'Jessica Jones. She was present when Peter Parker got bitten by that spider.' There is no inflexion in Sophie's voice, no expression in her eyes as she lifts her head and looks over the doctor's shoulder.

'Ah yes, Jessica Jones. I like her too.' He moves slightly to enable eye contact.

Sophie moves her head further to the right.

'Why do you like her, Sophie?'

He is beginning to annoy me. I know what he's doing: he's trying to engage my autistic daughter so he can check one of his boxes. *Engage with a person with a disability. Check. If it's an autistic person make eye contact. Check.*

I'm engaged in my negative thought-loop when Sophie makes eye contact with Dr Croft, and for the next five minutes she tells the story of Jessica Jones—of her adoption after her family were killed in an accident, of the super powers she developed after exposure to radiation. Sophie speaks in a shouted monotone, but she's having a conversation. Well, it's more of a monologue, really, but who cares? Dr Croft is smiling, animated, moving his arms and laughing with my daughter.

Something starts to crumble inside me. It's from the relief that someone is treating my daughter like a normal human being, and the joy that someone is being kind to her and not judgemental.

I savour the moment, before asking, 'How did you know Sophie likes Marvel?'

He looks at the floor and leans his elbows on his knees. 'I went through Sophie's history before you came in, and one of the nurses had sent me an email letting me know that Sophie used to carry a Marvel figurine with her every time she came in, so I've put it in her record under "hobbies".'

'Yup, love Marvel. Do you?' Sophie smiles and maintains eye contact with Dr Croft.

My happiness swells inside of me to the point I place a hand over my mouth so I don't let out a sob.

'Ah yes, I do,' he says. 'My son Peter loves it too—he's about your age.'

'Is he a skier as well?' I ask, nodding at the photos on the desk.

'No, he isn't. He stayed at home with his carers.'

The silence hangs heavy between us.

'Wonderfully neurodiverse, and very special,' Dr Croft adds, turning back to my daughter. 'Now, Sophie, how can I help you today?'

I'm too stunned to speak, shamed by self-pity. The shop assistant, Sophie's teacher and now Dr Croft were all, in fact, trying to help. The doctor's persistent kindness has somehow broken through my hardened shell of exhaustion and bitterness.

As we leave, Sophie looks straight at Dr Croft and shakes his hand. Outside the door, she smiles at me, grabs my hand and holds it tight.

We Do What We Can

Rukayatu Ibrahim

I see him as soon as I walk into the ward. His thin arms are protruding out of the stained, frayed, threadbare sheet that covers him on the bed. He is looking around the room; his eyes settle on me but do not meet my own. He looks away as I approach his bed.

I stand in front of the small, rusty steel frame. 'Good morning,' I say in Twi, the Ghanaian language common in this part of the country.

The young lady sitting by his bed, asleep in a rusty steel chair with no upholstery, jerks up. 'Huh?' she says, lifting her head and sitting up straight, squinting to look at me. She rubs her eyes, then fixes her scarf, which has come askew as she slept. 'Good morning,' she says.

'How is he doing?' I ask.

I look over at him again, and he is looking away, towards the other end of the room, at a group of people visiting a sick toddler in the corner. The toddler is crying between coughing spells.

'He is doing well,' she answers, looking at him too.

'Kofi, good morning,' I say, smiling.

He turns to look at me then. 'Good morning,' he says, not smiling.

'How're you?' I ask.

'I'm fine …' he says.

'He ate a little breakfast this morning and has not vomited again,' his mother says.

'That's good,' I say.

The bed adjacent to him holds two malnourished infants, sparse hair glistening on their scalps, skin hanging loosely on their skeletal bodies, blank stares on their faces. Their mothers are sleeping, heads down, arms around the babies, the rest of them slouched forward on their chairs.

'I'm just going to take a look and see how you're doing, okay?' I say to Kofi as I approach him and lift my stethoscope from around my neck.

He nods and lies flat on his back, placing his arms by his sides. I can tell he has done this many times and knows exactly what to do without being asked. His cheekbones stick out, and his big black eyes and long lashes appear more prominent on his thin, dark face.

I go through the motions of checking his mouth, listening to his heart and lungs. I then lift the stained hospital sheet and note the grossly distended, protruding abdomen, like that of a woman pregnant for nine months. The skin is taut over it, and there are multiple stretch marks. His abdomen glistens, and his umbilicus protrudes. I palpate carefully, looking at his face for pain, observing none. In the side of his abdomen there is a drain covered by a wet, serous-stained gauze. I follow the drain and note the clear fluid in the covered bowl it leads to, sitting on the floor under the bed. I measure the amount of fluid in the bowl and write it down in my folder. I check his genitals; the scrotal edema has improved.

I cover him up with the sheet again, thinking it is a shame that the hospital sheets are so old, so worn and ripped in places, with historic stains despite being sanitized. How much would it cost to have decent linen, I wonder?

His intravenous line leads to a plastic bag with *ceftriaxone* written across it, hanging on a rusty pole by the bed. I check his wrist to make sure the drip is working and his hand is not swollen.

'I'll be back with the team for rounds,' I say to his mother, who has been observing me from her seat the entire time.

'Yes, Doc,' she says.

I look again at the young boy in the bed and smile at him, meeting his eyes. He smiles back at me this time—a tired, thin, barely perceptible smile—then quickly looks away.

~

I check in on a couple more patients on my list, making sure my folders and plans are in order for rounds. I barely make it to the nurses' station in time.

Rounds are led by Dr Adongo, the head of the pediatric nephrology unit. He is not really a nephrologist, and there is no board-certified pediatric nephrologist in Ghana. He studied at the West African College of Physicians post-medical school, training to specialize in pediatrics. He has shadowed pediatric nephrologists in the USA, UK and Germany, and attended international pediatric nephrology conferences. He is a short, portly man with a big temper and a big belly—almost as big as that of some of his patients. He is infamous for bellowing on rounds, and trying to find fault with the examinations and treatment plans of house officers and medical students. We are all scared of him. He is, however, always very pleasant to patients and their families, as if to compensate for being horrible to his subordinates.

Today, there are three house officers (including me), seven medical students and an exchange student on the team. I am not sure where she's from, but she sticks out in the way the only Caucasian in a roomful of black people can. Her long blonde hair is in a ponytail, and her eyes are really blue. It scares me to look into them, I find. Perhaps I am not used to human beings with eye color that is not black or brown or whatever color black people's eyes are called.

Rounds start, and soon we are at Kofi's bedside. He ignores us, his mother still by his side. He closes his eyes, pretending to sleep, as one of the medical students presents his case. His mother watches us closely. I wonder what she is thinking, as she does not speak or understand English, the language we use on rounds.

'Kofi is a ten-year-old male with steroid-resistant nephrotic syndrome, also known as SRNS, admitted for worsening ascites, at risk for sepsis and hypertension,' the medical student begins.

He is tall and thin, wearing a clean, starched white coat over a long-sleeved shirt with a tie. He must be feeling hot, I think, as I stare at his dusty faux-leather shoes peeking out from under his well-ironed trousers. I am wearing a short white coat over a cotton African print dress, and I feel hot in this room with no air conditioner. The few ceiling fans do nothing to dispel the heat, but rather just rotate it around the heaviness of July's rainy season.

'This is his fifth hospital admission for ascites,' I hear the medical student say as I look over at Kofi again. He turns around in bed, his back to us. I wonder what he thinks of us and of this illness that he has lived with since he was five years old.

'What are his medications?' Dr Adongo yells at the medical student, who visibly shudders in response to this and flips aggressively through the papers on his clipboard, almost dropping it.

'He is on both lisinopril and losartan, aspirin, ceftriaxone, as well as furosemide.'

I come to the student's aid. 'He is also on a low-salt diet,' I add, knowing Dr Adongo will want to know that too.

The doctor goes on to quiz the medical student about the causes of nephrotic syndrome and its relation to ascites, the risk of sepsis in nephrotic syndrome and options for treatment in SRNS. The medical student, who has done his reading, mentions kidney biopsy, immunomodulators, dialysis or renal transplant if Kofi develops chronic kidney disease stage IV. The student has impressed Dr Adongo, who nods and pats him on the back, a rare occurrence. The doctor then asks me a few questions about lab results, vital signs and next steps, for which I have prepared. Soon, we're done and ready to move on.

The exchange student, who has been listening attentively with her head cocked to the side, raises her hand.

'Yes?' Dr Adongo asks.

'Has this patient had a kidney biopsy?' she asks, in what I recognize as an American accent.

'Pardon?' Dr Adongo yells, not understanding—probably due to her accent.

The rest of us smile and try to hide our laughter.

'Has he had a kidney biopsy?' she asks again, timidly.

Dr Adongo now appears to understand. He pauses, then asks, 'What is your name, and where are you from?'

'My name's Maggie, hi,' she says with a short, nervous laugh and small wave. 'I'm from the UCLA School of Medicine in Los Angeles, California, rotating here in pediatrics this month.'

'I see,' Dr Adongo responds, watching her with an eagle eye, sizing her up, perhaps deciding whether to terrorize her like he does us.

I smile to myself, wondering how he's going to handle this one.

'Good question, Maggie. You see, Maggie, for this patient to get a kidney biopsy, he will have to go to South Africa. We do not have the resources here for that.'

'Oh,' she says, seemingly bewildered. Her face turns red.

'As you know, South Africa is quite far from here, and it is expensive to fly there. Part of the reason this child is here again on admission is that his family cannot afford to buy him the medications to control his edema and hypertension. I do not think they can afford to go to South Africa for a kidney biopsy.'

Dr Adongo continues, 'I am sure your next question will be about genetic testing and whether we have tried any immunosuppressants or immunomodulators. We do not have genetic testing here. We can certainly draw the blood and have the lab send it to South Africa, but his family cannot afford to pay for it, and most immunomodulators are not available in Ghana at this time.'

Maggie's face turns redder, and she looks startled. 'Does insurance cover these … or charity care?'

Dr Adongo smiles broadly, all his huge, crooked white teeth showing. 'Insurance. Charity.' He nods emphatically as he says this. 'Very good concepts. Very, very good ideas.' He continues to nod. 'You see, Maggie, he does not have insurance. His family is not able to afford the small copay for the national insurance, which only pays for healthcare in this country and not for international testing or any healthcare outside the boundaries of this country. Charity is good too—very good, in fact—but we do not have any. Maybe you can give him charity, heh, Maggie? Maybe you can donate some money to send him to South Africa, heh?' He finishes loudly, smiling even more broadly. There are a few snickers.

Poor Maggie looks like she is about to cry.

Dr Adongo looks at her, and I sense something shift; he smiles at her in a way that is somewhat kind. As he moves away from the bedside, the medical team follows. 'We do what we can,' he says as he leaves. I stay back with Kofi and inform his mother that he'll be here for another couple of days as we try to decrease his ascites and control his blood pressure.

Kofi opens his eyes and stares at me as I say this. He looks as if he wants to ask a question, but does not. I wonder how much he understood of what just transpired. Unlike his mother, he goes to school and can speak and understand English. He looks downwards, tucks his hands under the sheet and draws the frayed edge up to his chest, staring across the room, watching the pediatric team as they walk away.

Blog of a Sick Girl

Emily Bourne

It was a normal Thursday; I'd just gotten home from school and spread myself across the sofa. My phone pinged to let me know my teacher had set homework, so I headed upstairs to grab my laptop. I sat down at my desk, opened my laptop and turned it on. The email read:

Class, I have set a piece of homework for Personal Development.
This one is a little bit different from what we usually do, but I think it will be an interesting topic to cover.
You have a week to plan and write a letter, to anyone of your choosing, to get something off your chest. It can be a personal letter, an opinion piece, a letter to the government, a letter to yourself . . .
This task is very subjective, meaning you can choose whoever you like and write about whatever you want. Each person's letter will be completely different.
If you have any questions, speak to me in class or by email.

After reading the email, I mulled over a multitude of possibilities. I didn't want to write to a family member or a celebrity. I wanted to try and get to the bottom of what makes each person different—and that's when the thought came to me. I started writing a blog.

DEAR STRANGER,

🕓 **January 1, 2015** ***Tags: Suffering, Pain, Relationships***

I've been struggling for a long time now. It's everything, all of it. Thinking back, it's hard to say when I was last truly happy.

I suffer every day, inside my body, inside my head. I have this thing wrong with me: I feel pain in my body all the time. Sometimes I can't move I'm in so much pain. I just look at the eyes of the boy who loves me and hope he will be enough to keep me here. I really hope.

I know he worries. He always tells me how he wouldn't know what he'd do if anything ever happened to me. I saw a piece he wrote (and before you judge me, I didn't intend to read something private) and the way he wrote was as if I'd die from the pain, and he was genuinely afraid. Me too.

My life has been turned upside down. No one means anything to me these days. People once close to me hate me now because of my 'bad attitude' (must be a coping mechanism, I guess).

I wish I hadn't lost everything. I wish I didn't feel the way I do. I don't give a shit what happens with my life from now on. I don't want a job; I don't want anything. I don't want. What happened to my life feels so unfair.

~

After writing that first post, I felt like a little bit of weight had been lifted from my shoulders. I was scared about printing it off and handing it in because nobody really knew about my chronic pain, and I didn't want them to mock me or look at me like I was some sick girl, or as if I was faking it.

A week passed, and my Personal Development lesson arrived. The teacher checked to see if we'd all completed our writing assignment but didn't make us hand them in—instead, she asked us what we'd learned from them. Some of my classmates had written to celebrities (Jameel had written to Kim Kardashian to thank her for her existence); some to parents who'd left; others to politicians, relatives or people in their life who'd died. The project, overall, taught us about ourselves (even Jameel, who realised how far his adoration for Kim Kardashian's ass would take him).

What had I learned? That writing helped me, a lot. I decided I would keep doing it.

WRITING AGAIN

🕓 **February 5, 2015; *Tags: Chronic Pain, Fibromyalgia, Summer Holidays***

At first, being diagnosed with chronic pain explained things, but it wasn't something about myself that was particularly important to me.

The back pain I'd experienced through periods of my life was because of a condition called fibromyalgia, so I was prescribed some tablets to alleviate the pain, and that's where I thought the story would end. For a while, I was coping with the pain, but it progressively got worse.

My first flare-up started last summer. I'd just started dating my first boyfriend, Adam, and within the month I was vomiting on his balcony at midnight. I was staying at home almost every day because I couldn't bear the heat. I was losing myself and my autonomy, bit by bit, each day.

I was sixteen and completely miserable. These days were supposed to be the best of my life, but each doctor's appointment gave me less hope, and with every 'maybe you'll grow out of this' I started to care less. It became harder to hear them through the pain that filled my body and thumped in my ears.

On a family holiday, I was barely able to hold up my own body.

DAYS THAT AREN'T TOO GOOD

🕓 **March 3, 2015; *Tags: Psychology, Psychiatry, Bravery***

Today at my mental health evaluation appointment, the psychologist asked how often I manage to get myself to college.

'Two or three days a week,' I said.

She wrote this down then asked me about what I do on days when I'm not feeling too good. I wasn't sure what to say. The truth is, I either lie on the sofa alone all day, or I go to my boyfriend's house. But I didn't want the psychologist to judge me, so I told her I always stay home.

She said, 'That must get lonely.'

What she didn't understand was that the story I told her is a sugar-coated version of my reality. I don't stay in my own home, lying on the sofa; I travel to my boyfriend's house, half-dead, in the cold and rain to sleep in his bed. Somehow, even though he isn't home, sleeping in his bed makes me feel less alone. Also, I'm sick of being a spectacle in my own house: being told to cheer up, to move on, like I'm not in pain all the time.

The psychiatrist asked if I ever have suicidal thoughts. I held my breath for a second, smiled, then shook my head: no. My heart raced, and I couldn't stop the tears that formed in my eyes. I let them roll down. She couldn't see what I was feeling if I refused to look at her. She told me that it's okay, that I'm brave. I wanted to tell her that I wish I didn't have to be.

RHEUMATOLOGY APPOINTMENT

🕓 **April 12, 2015; *Tags: Rheumatology, Adventure, Eating Disorder***

My heart broke when I heard my parents talk about me to my rheumatologist (I'm sixteen, but too vulnerable to go alone). My dad spoke about how I used to be quick-witted, engaged and always up for an adventure—and now he barely gets a word out of me, and I'm too tired to go exploring with him anymore.

My mum told the doctor how depressed I am and asked if there's anything he could prescribe. She told him I'd lost two stone because the pain I'm in makes it impossible to eat; the rheumatologist called this an eating disorder.

When he directed a line of questioning at me, I didn't know how to respond. All I wanted to do was cry. I didn't want any of this. If every day was going to feel like this, I didn't want them anymore, the days.

SMALL DETAILS

🕓 **May 12, 2015; *Tags: Conflict, Confusion, Chronic Pain***

Once there was a day when I got one small detail confused and messed up a whole lot of things. Someone important to me said I was manipulative and calculated. When I asked what they meant, they told me I knew exactly what I had done. But I had no idea.

I only realised the mistake when they explained the situation to me. I'd confused two bits of information—a common symptom for people with chronic pain. They thought I'd done this deliberately to get what I wanted. My heart had never felt heavier. Is that really how they saw me?

I'd never felt worse; I was just trying to cope. I was trying my best but fucked that up.

They told me to 'stop it with the waterworks', as if I could stop crying while being told that they didn't recognise me anymore, that no one enjoyed being around me—as if I was enjoying a life full to the brim of suffering.

Sometimes my mind goes back to that day, and I always get palpitations. I don't think I'll ever let go of everything I felt then.

All I needed was to hear, 'I believe you.'

SOMETIMES

🕓 **June 9, 2015; *Tags: Hearing, Seeing, Sick***

Sometimes I struggle to hear what people are saying and need to put captions on the TV, because the pain is too loud.

Sometimes I need to close my eyes because it physically hurts to see.

Sometimes I can't enjoy eating because of the pain.

Sometimes smelling things immediately makes me feel (or be) sick or causes a migraine.

BREAKFAST

🕓 **July 10, 2015; *Tags: Crumpets, Tea, Progress***

Today I woke up early and made breakfast. It wasn't a big meal, just some crumpets with marmite. And a cup of tea (one sugar, lots of milk). I had to take breaks, and force the food down, but I got there eventually.

Tomorrow, I'll try to do the washing-up too.

FORGIVENESS

🕓 **December 9, 2015; *Tags: Memories, Healing, Forgiveness***

I'm sorry if it's hard for you to read this, but I need to stop carrying this burden around in my heart. I need to take control of these memories. I need to let them go. I know you didn't mean to hurt me. These posts are about me being able to heal, not directing any hatred on you.

I love you and I forgive you. I hope you can forgive me.

HEALING IN PROGESS

🕓 **January 1, 2017; *Tags: Final Post, Progress, Healing***

This is going to be my last post. I originally wrote these entries to help myself, but I am finally ready to let them go. Although we've never met, stranger, I wish you all the best. Thank you for taking some of the burden from me. I hope these posts have also helped you to overcome issues that you're dealing with.

Here are some things I've learned about healing over the past couple of years:

- It isn't linear; you have to start over again and again, and that's okay.
- It doesn't make the damage disappear; it just means it can't have control over you anymore.
- It isn't always pretty—you will need to ugly cry it out sometimes.
- It's hard to reflect upon yourself, and to be alone. These days we fill our lives with so many *things* that we rarely have the time for either.

~

Today is a Tuesday.

Tuesdays are my therapy days. My therapist teaches me how to cope; she lets me talk to her until the sun goes down, and she holds my hand through it all.

Today I ask if I can stay a little longer, and she replies, 'Take all the time you need.'

Fuddle

Vanessa McClelland

They come to you first in your dreams. Images losing their footholds on reality. Dripping faces. Wavering borders. Imperfect fiction. You take it as a bad meal. A typical dreamscape. In the morning, the filaments of the abstractions coloring your dreams dry up in the light of day. You forget about them. Life moves on, as it does. The sun rises. You go to work. The sun falls. Then you go to bed and dream in unreality.

You repeat this. For days. Your nights are somehow never quite restful, never fulfilling the eternal promise of relaxation and recharge. Instead they're full of toil.

Your boss worries about you. It's nothing, you say. Probably coming down with the flu. It's written off. Swept under the rug.

Until they emerge from your subconscious's vault. Dashes and smears and little scampering motes come and go before your eyes. Come and go. Like dead skin cells on the surfaces of your eyeballs. You focus on one, then it's gone. Another dances at the edge until you focus again, then that disappears. Vanishes.

They're only ghosts at first. You dismiss them as a fancy, an overactive imagination, stress. That's all it is, just an element of the world out *there* invading the world in *here*.

~

It's early morning. You're brushing the sugar from your teeth after your breakfast of multicolored cereal. Your reflection shimmers in the mirror. Leaning forward, you squint; toothpaste foam decorates your lips. It's not the mirror that shimmers, but the edges of your reflection. It blurs. And then smears, as though some child has dipped a finger in your face and dragged it across the glass like it was crafted from wet paint.

The edges drip and drag.

Blinking, you try to discern if you're awake or still in one of your dreams that are not quite restful and not quite dreams. The rabbit in your chest thumps and thumps, and everything along the edges of your vision goes fuzzy. Not the weird illusions you're seeing, but a real effect. Your vision tunnels and pinpoints to a tiny black dot.

When you wake up, there's a goose egg on your head and a small blood spatter on the tile. And the smears have blurred everything around you.

~

You let the panic wash over you. You squat in the tub for hours. It provides a bulwark against the smudged world pressing in and in and in. The indistinct edges don't appear to be harming you, but they are there, insidious, changing everything from what it once was to this blurry impressionist drug trip, without the drugs.

You try the optometrist first, though your gut says the problem is not with your vision. The doctor listens as you explain the blurred edges and the blended colors and the smears. Smears everywhere. The doctor nods as you talk, and you watch invisible fingers drag colors through her face, twisting her eyes around, drawing out her nose to something an anteater could use.

She tries multiple lenses, testing your vision as you read lines from a board across the room through the glass. She puffs air on your eyes. Your vision is fine, and she kindly suggests a therapist's office nearby.

Reasonable enough. You make an appointment.

The therapist listens as you once again explain the blurred edges and the smears, the fuzziness that isn't due to any corneal malfunction. You've given a name to this ocular effect: the fuddles. And you wonder if it makes you more … *off* now you've named the phenomena.

Your mind still feels sharp, you explain. You can continue the work in your consulting office. You can answer the game-show questions. You can sing the lyrics to all your favorite songs. Other than the smears, the smudged appearance of things, you don't feel affected.

The doctor prescribes a drug. You ask, 'So soon?' He says it should help with your delusions. The smudged-out eyes of the doctor don't look like delusions to you, though your mind argues that this is not normal.

You go home. You take the drug. When you wake up, you feel all smeared inside.

~

You have faith in modern medicine, and you continue taking the medication per the doctor's orders. Perhaps it will get better, you think, as the walls between you and the world lose their focus. You get up from bed, move from the room. Walk outside. Move again. Pieces of you feel left behind, detached, smudged away and lost. Sometimes your singularity returns, your body and being crisp again, and sometimes the fuddles work hard to keep you amorphous.

The fuddles. What are they? What do they want? Why do they want to trick you, make you think the world is a lie?

After a night where you nearly disintegrate and float away, you accept the medication isn't working. You tell your doctor. It gives the fuddles power over me, you explain. So you try another medication and another.

One of them withholds sleep, and you're up late following the rabbit hole of internet links into mental illusions and evil energies. In a flashing ad, there's the address for a local psychic who specializes in spirit banishment and Catholic-style exorcisms.

You've tried everything else. The world is smeared and smudged and mussed as if by childish fingers. You've *tried* everything *else*.

You call the psychic to set an appointment. It's 3 a.m.

~

The consult goes smoothly. You tell the psychic about the smears and the blurs and the long smudges destroying the straight and even order of the world around you, how something—the fuddles—have rearranged everything, you think for their sick, twisted amusement. And that only *you've* noticed.

It's a story you've explained so many times.

The psychic nods and listens, and you're reminded of the optometrist and the therapist. You explain it all, clear as day: what you see now isn't what you used to see. Everything has changed, and you're completely aware it's changed, and you still feel in control. You see what the fuddles are doing—perhaps they're malevolent spirits—and they, well, they're mocking you, making sure you see them, enjoying the twists and turns they have constructed in your mind. How they're making you so *unsure*. They like it.

The psychic nods some more, heartfelt and understanding. She tells you all about earth spirits, local spirits, and spirits of the dead. You listen, but none of it sounds similar to the fuddles. You think she's talking out of her ass, which feels very disrespectful since you're the one the seeing unaccountable things.

You think of them as illusions, since you know they can't be real.

The psychic gives you a chant to repeat, and burns some candles and sage, and tells you to perform a cleansing ritual every night between the full moon and the new. Your heart's not in it, but you try because you're desperate. You're tired of the smeared faces and dripping buildings and trees with wriggly lines. You're tired of the façade all around you.

You're ready for something real. You burn the sage, chant the words and splash some protection water over your eyes before you sleep at night.

Your dreams are a van Gogh of colors and swirls, and nothing is as it should be. When the moon is new, the fuddles should be banished, the psychic said. But after the darkest night, after you wake up from your infested dreams, you blink at your ceiling and see finger-painted swirls of browns and greens and mustard yellow. They remind you of a mold infestation.

The fuddles smear the lines and blur the colors.

Fine. Two can join this battle.

~

At the craft store you buy a canvas, an easel and an array of colors, bright and dark, shades from nature, all singing authenticity.

That first day after the new moon, you begin. You set up your easel in the spare room and grab a brush and stare at the window, at the off edges, the bent frame, the fingerprints of the fuddles. With your tool of choice, you copy what you see in a rough, untrained hand. You paint the window frame in bold, bright oak lines, struggling to make them straight and proportionate, and you make the thick blackout curtains, currently a pale purple—a color you'd find in an Easter basket—dark and heavy. You paint the window for hours, focusing on what it looked like when it was *real*, before the fuddles decided to bend your perception. You paint it like it should be. You paint *reality*.

When you are done, the oil colors are thick on the canvas, wet and glistening under the ceiling light. The straight lines draw you in. Against all expectations, they are actually straight and clean. You nearly sob. *Straight lines.*

Your breath is shaky as you smear the painting with your right index finger. If this is what you want, I give it to you, you chant, using your own words instead of the holy prayer the psychic gave you. You drag your finger over the fresh painting, drawing divots through the paint, curling it around—then, with a sharp drop, yanking it over the edge of the canvas. Paint speckles the floor.

You take all five right-hand fingertips and squiggle them across the window you painted, spinning chaos and uncertainty in the credible image you created, making it something fuddle-like. You lay your palm on the splattered canvas and press down, feeling paint squish out along the edges.

Chaos. You are creating chaos.

When you finish, you turn your back on the image and you wash in the bathroom and you climb into bed. Eyes closed, you take in deep, methodical breathes, like your therapist suggested. You continue the prayer, now something more fervent, invoking the name of God, begging for a resolution to this haunting.

Still begging, you pass into sleep. They visit your dreams. You wake up resigned.

In your bedroom, the lines are smeared. You climb from a bedlam of curves and smudged borders that make up your bed, then grab your robe, pulling on the blurred garment. You brush your teeth, drink some water and feel a twisting knot growing and tightening and swelling in your belly. You can't keep doing this. It's pecking away at your stability. *Peck. Peck. Peck.*

Thinking of your painting, you go into the temporary studio. A gasp escapes you.

The window. The window of your room is solid. The real window is *real*, with lines that are straight and glass that doesn't droop and black blackout curtains, and there are no swipes smudging the perfection of the truth of it.

You drop to your knees and truly sob. Cry in relief and in hope and in some uncontrollable release of all the terror of a future you'd almost resigned yourself to live through. Minutes pass as you stare at the window—at the one perfect object surrounded by imperfection.

You go to your painting. You've left it a mess, destroyed the classic precision of it. But today the painted window is smeared and smudged and blurry around the edges in a way that isn't exactly what you created. Leaning in, you spot a divot in the image drawn long, like a finger has slid through the viscous coating that's almost dry after an evening of airing out: a finger has fuzzed up the glass, making an impression.

Perhaps the fuddles just needed their own place, you think magnanimously, though at a deeper level you hope you've created a trap, that you have captured them in the paint.

It's yours, you tell the fuddles aloud. It's all yours.

The rest of your house remains fuddled. You prepare another canvas.

Does He Feel Warm?

Al Campbell

In the room next to Teddy's is a newborn. A boy. Frail, it goes without saying. He lies on his chest in a clear box. Tubes run through him, and sticky sensors measle him, as they do Teddy, but miniature versions. I hear one of the many doctors declare that the child is diabetic, 'among other things.' When these Other Things are discussed, voices in that room dial down. The mother is asked at least once a day if her pregnancy was routine. *Yes*, she answers, less shocked than offended. *This is the first I've heard about anything.* Her husband arrives, tall, well dressed. Husband and wife wear rings that cannot be unnoticed. The newborn has a sister, blonde, aged perhaps four or five. *Indie.* Billboard-pretty, his family.

I wish I knew his name; I never hear it spoken, but I know he will have a surgery tomorrow, more in the coming weeks. The couple is worried about the effects of the general anaesthetic. The surgeon tries to reassure them but says something like, *That's the least of our worries at present*, then leaves. With a laugh. A doctor's laugh, one quite relaxed in its own company, even as it rips through the blue-white belly of the ward. He clip-clops away down the corridor, his glossy black clogs like hooves.

Six p.m., and the parents turn on the news in their son's room. The volume is absurd, unnerving, the faux-fawning voices—*Back to you, Ray. Thanks so much, Tamsin*—thrashing their way along the floor. The dissonant hoot and chaff of the Bunnings and banking commercials pitch me to my feet. Kissing Teddy's forehead—the only part of his face not vandalised by clamps and valves and tape—I tell the nurse I'm going for a walk. He nods. The room is tight and mechanised, grimly purposed. His job is to patrol, refill, adjust. Mine is to watch and wait. I know it's a relief to be free of me.

~

Me, trying to slot a nugget of dry, untouched cereal between Teddy's ziplocked lips. Back when he used his mouth to eat. 'Not hungry, Teddy Bear? Not like you.' My hand against his forehead, then tapping twice on his water cup. 'Drink up, big Ted.'

Teddy mimicked my two taps on the cup's lid, lifted it to his mouth, drank.

Breezing into the kitchen—freshly showered, fizzing with blue-chip cologne—Jerrik ruffled Teddy's ringlets. 'How goes it, Egghead? Sleep well?'

Teddy laughed and looked up from his iPad, a *7.30 Report* clip from 2004. Grabbing his father's hand, he ran the back of it gently under his chin, back and forth, relaxed and affectionate. With his free hand he reached up to caress Jerrik's ears.

I asked Jerrik, 'Do you think he feels warm?'

Jerrik mumbled, 'Warm?' Windsor-knotting his tie.

But a switch was flicked. 'Yes, *warm!* You know—the opposite of *cool*? Do you think he feels *warm*?' Less a switch of late than a rogue, sparking fuse.

Teddy waggled his empty cup above his head.

Hands falling to his sides, Jerrik gave me one of his *I-don't-know-what-you-want-me-to-do* looks. 'Take his temperature if you're worried,' he told the tie.

I picked up Teddy's iPad, leaned into his space. 'Looking at Mum,' I said, lightly guiding his face—mellow, expressionless—to mine. 'Use your words, Ted. Tell me what you want.'

After opening his communication app, Teddy's fingers darted across the screen with the touch of a safecracker. 'I. Want. More. Water. Please. Mummy,' said Liam, the pre-programmed 'young male Australian' voice. Teddy placed the iPad in his lap, threaded his fingers through mine. He squeezed. I squeezed back. We did this for a minute, maybe more, before his focus returned to the YouTube search pane and I was dismissed. He typed *The Mikado.*

'Good talking, Teddy boy,' I said.

'Thank. You,' said Liam, as Teddy scrolled through related searches for Gilbert and Sullivan.

~

Paediatric intensive care is all light, all white, all glass. A whole floor of frostbite. I glance into the baby's room as I slide Teddy's door closed.

In his box, the infant is panting, doing his best to breathe, but the faces of his mother and father tilt up at the leering television, reverential as though heeding a prophet. Their eyes never turn from the screen, even as words jab and ping between them: *protest*, *highway*, *hamburger*, *ute*. Indie sits on the floor with her father's big phone, ensorcelled as a kitten with a ball of yarn.

The Other Things are newborn too. I see them nestling close to the tiny boy, their breath butcher-red.

~

Mrs Redman calling from school. Teddy's fine, she said, doing his work, always a lovely boy. 'But it's lunchtime and he's lying on the ground, no interest in playing. He could hardly wait for break time once, always first to the swings. But he's been like this all term. I'm getting a bit worried.'

'All term?' I said. 'I'll come and collect him. Do you think he feels warm?'

An hour later: 'A growing boy,' said the GP, with a poke at Teddy's knee. 'Just dropping some puppy fat, aren't you, mate?' Teddy wiped the unexpected touch from his skin. 'Headaches, body pain?'

'That's the problem,' I said. 'It's so hard to know.'

'Baby Panadol,' smiled the doctor, with a comforting pat on my arm.

Teddy was down five kilos.

~

I sit on a bench in the walkway, just inside the doors of the secured ward. On the walls, fairy lights and children's art, a welcome change from the panels of panic-red electrical sockets in Teddy's room here. Twenty-seven in all. Twenty-seven glum little faces.

A nurse approaches, hesitates, moves on. I know her from 10A. Teddy spent weeks in ante-roomed isolation (just in case), tests pending, everyone but us robed, gloved, masked. And they know me, the staff, know to avoid me. Know just as well to assume things are in hand. A nasogastric feed every three hours, around the clock. His vomit expertly cleaned up. Daily cares: teeth, hair, bath, sheets—check. Biopsy sites cleaned and dressed. Every drop relinquished by his bladder, every peristaltic crinkle of his bowel—the all-important, under-surveillance bowel—recorded, spreadsheeted (time/volume/colour; blood Y/N; mucus Y/N; discomfort on a scale of one to ten.)

Unlikeable, that Mrs … *whatever.* Demanding, yes. But better a prickly parent who does the donkey work than a charmer with her feet up.

Around a corner, two new mothers, one sobbing: *They say she'll walk, one day, probably. She's definitely vision-impaired. As for all the other things … too early to tell.*

But I know the mother won't have long to wait. Other Things grow unfairly fast.

~

'So unfair, these new regulations,' said Jerrik, calling at 2 a.m. 'Burying us in red tape.' He was so sorry.

Teddy had only just drifted off to sleep, agitated and fussy. His low-grade fever came and went. Oddly, he kept asking for food—*I. Want. More. Sandwich. Please. Mummy*—only to spit out what he'd chewed. He looked thinner, but I couldn't know for sure; he wouldn't stand still on a scale.

Mindful of Teddy, I whispered into the phone. 'Someone staying behind to give you a hand?' It was not a genuine question.

Silence.

'Didi? Kiki? Loulou?'

When he answered, Jerrik's defiant tone was like a slap. 'Minnie.'

'Goodness,' I said, too tired for tone. I wasn't sure why I even answered. 'Up to the M's already?'

Earlier this afternoon: 'Something viral,' the GP had said.

'Like I told you, it'll pass. Try some pain relief. Will he take baby Panadol?'

'No, he won't, not once in the ten years you've treated him.'

'But it's yummy. Kids love it.'

'Not my kid,' I had snapped. 'Read his file, why don't you?' I'd left the door open, then charged back down the corridor to slam it.

I was about to relay this to Jerrik, but he was gone, had either hung up or dropped out.

I didn't try calling him back.

~

It's 6.20 p.m. I stay benched in the corridor, trusting my child doesn't die while I'm out here, dodging the sports report, the Southern Oscillation Index, listening instead to a young mother's tears, and to the silence of another who can't possibly know what to say.

This is her first baby, her only baby, the one who might walk, who might see, who might not. As the new mother speaks, her hands skim her belly—an exhausted, postpartum sag. A lonely, liminal place no longer shared yet not quite her own, where something routine went amiss, whose soundness will always be suspect, queried. Quietly blamed.

I wish I could talk her through it: that day when she finally takes her child home and notices the leak in her ceiling. It will be in a room far down the hall, a spare room for storage, overnighters. She'll place a bucket under the leak to catch the drips.

In the next downpour the leak will become urgent, because the drips have more heft. The bucket fills quickly. She'll buy one that is bigger, then another, then more. Her baby's father will try to patch it, but that only makes it worse. The carpet is ruined. Crusty brown mould cankers the ceiling. It leaks even when it's not raining.

One night during a storm, the young mother will get up on a stepladder, press a baby blanket to the leak. It soaks through and she will throw it to the floor, get another, one that is thicker, then a towel, a blanket. Soon she'll have emptied the linen cupboard. She will tape plastic to the ceiling, but the tape won't hold. The whole roof sways with damp.

Before long the house is flooded, water ankle-deep. Furniture floats, table legs ooze and buckle.

One day, desperate, she'll hold her mouth to the leak, and swallow.

With her lips to the ceiling she won't know if it's day or night. She'll decide it doesn't matter. Nothing else will be done—no cakes baked, no playdates, everything stamped *overdue.* No time for more children; the mother dares not leave the drip. Her jaw will ache, and her child will cry, but she'll stay focused, her mouth open, swallowing, swallowing. It's the only thing that works, more or less. The only thing that stops her family being swept away. The leak will be all she consumes, other appetites gone. Her husband and the years will scatter.

People will check on her, from time to time, in the room far along the hall. They'll praise her, her composure and strength. They'll see she's no longer unmoored, as once she was, her bloated blue lips now fused with the ceiling, her feet with the rusted tiers below. They'll see she no longer frets about fixing the leak, no longer waits for the day when she'll climb down from the ladder.

'We'll see ourselves out,' her visitors will wave, 'cheery bye.' Everyone so relieved, none will notice the Other Things, how they've claimed the house as their own. How their flickering, pinprick eyes hunt the halls, deciding who may leave and who may not. 'Cheery bye,' call the visitors who glide by the rippling pelts, wet and slick against the walls, seeing only ulcered paint. Hearing not the red roars of triumph, only the skirling screams of a bird.

~

Another early evening, weeks ago. Teddy and I, lying on his bed—a single, but space enough to lie nose to nose. There was a fog. Impenetrable. Through the windows we could see precisely nothing, blindfolded by a meaty ghost-grey felt. We were like specimens, a giant mournful face pressed to our glass jar.

Jerrik called. Everyone was stranded at the office, too dangerous to be on the roads. Not that anyone was doing much; all eyes were glued to it, tongues tuned to it—rarer, all agreed, than an eclipse. This city of tropical monotony usually sees no such fogs. Jerrik would have to stay put. Might as well roll up his sleeves. So sorry.

'What if we were to run outside, Ted?' I said. 'Hold out our arms, let ourselves disappear?' Fall backwards into the warm grey glug. Tag along when it shipped out.

Teddy sat up, amazed, perhaps afraid.

'It's only your lucky star,' I told him, 'its great lantern eyes dull and sad because you're poorly.'

He waved at the fog, blew a kiss—an open-palmed double-clunk against his chin, lips curled in, an inverse pucker. Nobody blows kisses like Teddy.

Lying down again, he set his chin delicately in the whorl of my ear, held it there for minutes on end. Our fingers laced, he squeezed, I squeezed, back and forth we went. I don't know if it brings him some kind of relief or sensory feedback, or if it's simply something we do. His body simmered, his temperature back up, his skin the colour of sucked-over bones. He smelled hollow. I opened a story, but he closed the book at once, put it back on the pile by his bed, resettled his chin on my ear.

We both slept a little, until something kicked open my eyes, dragged its claws down my face, doing its job—feeding fear, ruining rest.

Teddy stayed the week in his room, a few dry crackers every other day.

'Some viruses can hang around,' said the GP, 'but let's take some urine. Has a dentist had a look? Could be an abscess?'

Three nights later, Teddy sat for an hour on the toilet, red-faced with straining, as he produced a dribble of urine and a bowl full of blood.

Twelve years old, twelve kilos gone, and we were off to hospital.

~

Hospitals, two of them once upon a time, either side of a feted river. Bountiful care for our flush-faced children, choice for their hand-wringing parents, the dreaded, diddling ferryman unfrocked. 'But less is So-Much-More,' they swore to us, our civic custodians, collapsing two into one—this frost-fortressed realm—promising epic *specialist* care, *gold standards* and *best practice*, oracles of wisdom and healing. We, the parents, pitiful and panicked, shrugged. What did we care? Wisdom and healing—all we want, after all.

And so began the ferryman's sly reprise, casting us off, Teddy and I, across a roiling stygian marsh, sworn oaths triaged to oblivion. Before us, a bastard-beast: heads atop thick serpentine necks, a snarl of junkyard dogs erupting from its middle. Its many baked-black mouths and rows of arrowed teeth chomp the air at our throats. Behind us, the whirlpool of wards, those dismal hovels, double-doored and pathogen-flushing (just in case). Yet the price of safe passage is not our pennies, but our hands above our heads.

Scans, scopes, bloods and dyes. Fifteen kilograms and falling.

Biopsies shall tell us more. A raven, reading from a note tied around its leg. It has oars instead of wings. A hopeless half-bird.

'Is my son dying?'

We don't think *ssssso*, hisses something soft and gilled below my feet. *But he* izzzzz *in trouble, if that'sss any help.*

Tiny capsuled eyes crawl the darkest verticils of my son's failing body. *What is hard to see is harder to fix*, they caution.

Gut-related? froths one of the heads, its foul breath squirting like lanced disease.

I'm thinking immuno, foams another, *since I'm a rheumo.*

The brain? The pituitary?

These lymph nodes, let me at them!

Clinically insignificant! growl three sets of jaws.

But the ELECTROLYTES! spits a chorus. *Anyone heard of a REFEED?*

Thirty kilos—half of Teddy—gone. Immediate intubation, their only point of agreement. Exclusive enteral nutrition via a percutaneous endoscopic gastrostomy.

Nourish him, at least. A synchronised nod.

Doing nothing takes time. Another pod-nod. *Deciding nothing takes time.* The heads don't like to be hurried.

'But,' I challenge, my voice a gasp, too low to the ground; voices of the mortal and medically unconsecrated atrophy fast in this burred, blasted air, 'his sensory issues …? A feeding tube …? You know he'll fight it. Teddy won't understand.'

Let us tell you how hospitals work, roars one of the dogs, a bucking ram between its jaws.

'This is so extreme,' I cry, hands still raised, shoulders welded by ache. 'Shouldn't diagnosis be the priority?'

It's care our way, *or care withdrawn, Mrs—, Mrs—*, bellows the beast. *Without it, he DIES!*

The heads weave and whir around me, so close they clot into one. *Up to you, you're the mother. Up to you! You're the mother! YOU'RE THE MOTHER!*

The sculptures that hang above us—giant wooden parrots, award winners with eyeless, tumescent heads—begin to multiply. Suddenly, thousands of them twitch to life, the gullet of the building choked by a blind, convulsant swarm.

Everything falls silent as a creature emerges from the rear, as wide as it is long, its face beaked, heads and hands bog-green, a writhing jumble of tails and horns haemorrhaging behind it. It hover-hops over dunes of dying, dismembered bulls.

I see myself reflected in its many eyes, a grotesque of mirrors that diminish me—ever older and smaller—until I disappear, leaving Teddy behind, alone, his hand held out to no one.

A clipboard is thrust at my face. *Sign here*, it says, its voice stilling the currents.

~

I return to my son. The news is over, Indie and her parents gone, quiet restored. The baby boy sleeps in his box. As expected, the Other Things have grown since I left. The litter sits up now, little claw-buds blooming. One licks the child's ear, getting a taste of him. The others cast long shadows along his butter-soft body, waiting for the parents—whom they've come for, after all—to return.

Doctors consult outside Teddy's room. Heads huddle over

monitors, scanning results, straightening up to talk, hushed, furtive. I track the skin on their faces—how it moves, where their eyes rest—and count the clicks of their pens, observe how long their knuckles squirm in airless pockets, grappling with their godliness revoked.

They don't know. They truly don't know.

I spend days this way, and I can't say what frightens me more: a hospital confounded, or the Other Things born alongside my own baby, here with us, lurking at home too, watching us always, day and night, as we lie nose to nose, chin to ear. So monstrous now, a flick of a tail cracks me like an egg. So cruel, they glue the broken shell of me back together.

Teddy's cheek is soft, cooling, his fever finally outplayed.

I pick up his hand, lace our fingers, and wait.

You Have Dysentery

Leah Baker

I walk out of the hospital into the hot Indian night. A few blocks east, I come to the alley I've been directed to. At the end of the long dark corridor, I see the blue light of an ATM. I need cash to pay a hospital bill, and this is the only path. Cows line the shadowy passage, chewing noisily on trash. Their large bodies move slowly, a faint white glow reflecting off their hides in the dimness.

A snarling stray dog erupts out of the gloom, and I leap back, screaming.

It is not aiming for me, but for one of the cows. The two animals battle over a scrap or a plastic bag, I can't see which. I want to flee, but I have to get the money.

I am in Varanasi, the oldest continuously inhabited city in the world, considered one of the holiest sites in India. The city was built around the Ganges. To bathe in this river is a sacred act. Thousands gather daily at the eighty-four ghats of Varanasi: stone steps along the riverbank. When a Hindu person dies, it is an honor for them to be cremated on the ghats then pushed into the water, covered in white cloth and surrounded by marigold blooms the sacred color of saffron. Here, the living can be ferried onto the water by a boatman to witness the incineration of corpses. Here, you may pay a child in exchange for a paper boat with a single candle in it, to be immolated as you set it out on the water: a symbolic prayer. Here, you may watch roaming cattle and stray dogs feast at the riverbank on the piles of bones of those who have passed.

The holy water of the great Ganges is therefore filled with death: ashes of cremated bodies, sewage both human and animal, and soil from the thousands who bathe in it daily.

~

I arrived in Varanasi on a train with my traveling partner, Brian. The rail system is its own startling entity. We fought against a bustling line of hundreds for our tickets. We took an overnight rail.

Brian started to feel unwell on the train. In India, when you defecate in the train's squat-toilet bathroom, the waste is released onto the tracks below, contributing to a unique smell of incense, burned plastic, pollution, urine and raw sewage.

We woke to the sound of the chaiwallah calling out his familiar mantra, *'Chai-ii, chai-ii, garam chai-ii'*, as he passed through the crowded, narrow rows of sleeper beds, serving up his special sugary tea.

Brian was sick in the railway bathroom when we arrived. He took a course of Cipro, an antibiotic that most travelers in developing countries keep on hand in case of an intestinal infection. We waited to see if it would cure his ailment—it didn't. He was sick all night in the tiny room we were renting. He was losing fluid fast. I stole bottles of water out of the boxes in the guesthouse lobby, as no one was there to take my rupees at that hour.

His temperature soared. He sweated. He hallucinated.

In the morning I decided we must go to a hospital. We took a rickshaw across town but had to walk the rest of the way when the driver realized how sick Brian was. Rickshaw drivers have a superstition that if someone dies in their carriage, they have to purchase a new one. We were dumped out to walk along the street, though Brian could barely progress. He leant on me for support. He was a ghost of thread and wire. We had to stop often. People laughed and pointed upon seeing this tall, sick foreign man being led around by a smaller foreign woman.

Entire families lay in packed rows outside the hospital, at the entrance, and inside the waiting room, mostly on the floor. Because we could pay for it, we only had to wait a few hours to be admitted into the emergency section: a small, windowless room filled with hard cots inhabited by patients sicker than Brian. As I had during much of my time traveling through this country, I felt my own privilege with stark embarrassment that spread across my cheeks hotly.

Once Brian was admitted, I fought to receive service from every counter at the hospital. I was volleyed back and forth. When I visited a counter for the third or fourth time to demand that Brian receive a laboratory test, the receptionist slapped my hand, which was resting on the desk. This wasn't the first time I'd been slapped on the hand in India; the other time had been in an airport, when I'd asked what time our delayed flight would arrive.

My voice had never sounded so loud and so sure as it did in the hospital, yet I felt so small and so unsure. I had to take a rickshaw to purchase IV bags in a pharmacy across town. I had to deliver Brian's stool sample to the lab for testing—a sample so watery that it was mistaken for urine.

None of the doctors were washing their hands between patients; they also didn't wear gloves. I asked one of them to wash his hands before inserting an IV, but I noticed there was no soap at the small, dirty metal sink.

Some of the people in the room were dying.

Around one in the morning, Brian and I were asked to leave the hospital to make room for more patients. But first we'd have to pay for the services—in cash. 'There's an ATM down the street,' said the receptionist.

~

When I reach the ATM, I see immediately that it is defunct. Wires hang out where buttons used to be, and the screen flickers.

A man on a motorcycle drives up to use the ATM. His face looks as disappointed as mine does. I ask him if he knows of another ATM. He does, but it is far. He gestures behind him and tells me to get on.

I climb onto the back of this stranger's motorcycle. We ride past angry dogs, cows, through alleyways. When we arrive at the ATM, I try to tip him profusely for the ride, but he refuses.

Around three in the morning, I leave the hospital with Brian. I break into a sweat in the humid night air, while he erupts into a fit of cold shivering. I have never witnessed shaking like this before. His chest and neck are speckled with what look like hives, and I sit him down on the dirty pavement. He convulses. His teeth chatter violently. Perhaps it is a reaction to the cold fluid running through his veins from the IV, or perhaps it's his fever breaking.

On the slow walk back to the guesthouse, we pass hundreds of sleeping people along darkened ghats. They are thin and impoverished. The only waking person is a man in a boat out on the Ganges, who hollers at us.

This walk is one of the eeriest experiences of my life. I am not sure if I believe in ghosts, but if I did, I wouldn't be able to comprehend the number of spirits that have been released in this longstanding cremation ground.

I again feel the sharp embarrassment of my obscene privilege. Here I am, a healthy woman walking with a man who just had his life saved because we could afford it. Meanwhile, the ghats are filled with homeless people sleeping on the hard ground.

~

The next day, I call the hospital repeatedly to receive the lab results: 'Dysentery.'

When I was a girl, I used to play the computer game *Oregon Trail* on one of those Macintosh PCs with the small, square, black screens. When a character in the game got dysentery, *YOU HAVE DYSENTERY* would appear in pixelated white text. Nine times out of ten, that character would die.

Brian's prescribed medication works within the next forty-eight hours, although it takes him months to recover completely. He rescues me from a monkey attack later that week, and cares for me a month later when I fall ill on a trek in the isolated Himalayan region of Ladakh. There is no hospital. There are no roads. Brian carries my pack when we cross the highest pass, because I am buckling under its weight. The wind whips my face. I have to stop and catch my breath between each step because the air is so thin. We are surrounded by snow, wandering yaks, donkeys, Ladakhi shepherds, and Buddhist stupas at which I pray that I do not die.

~

When I return to the USA after my time abroad, I'm hardened. I've been away for more than a year. My body is different. The hardships of my relationship with Brian outweigh its strength. I leave him and my heart aches. I go to see healers. I stay in an apartment that is empty except for an air mattress and my bicycle. One of my colleagues remarks loudly that I 'look a little damaged'.

While Brian recovered in our guesthouse in the week that followed our trip to the hospital, I took many silent walks along that river of death. I came across a mural of the goddess Akhilandeshvari on a large column. Her name means 'one who is never not broken' and she sits boldly astride a crocodile.

I don't think breaking experiences such as this damage us. I feel more full, grateful, mature and courageous than when I left.

The Shaking Man

Reinfred Dziedzorm Addo

For Terri Beamer Shelor, Karen Gaines, Rebecca Blackert Epperly and Kristin King

Part I

I met the shaking man in London Town. In a red Tube cab, my eyes were glued to the movements of his hands, ticking, repetitive. I made nothing of it, and three days later serendipity united us in the gray, wide building of my Shoreditch clinic.

He was marching in place at the rehabilitation gym, seeming to tremble from the exertion of lifting feathery weights wrapped around his ankles. As I slowly recalled where we'd first met, I looked closely at the shaking man and saw that his buzzing had become more pronounced. He was quivering.

I immediately understood, and he confirmed it himself two weeks later: *tremors*. They had started a year-and-yesterday ago, he told me, and upon medical counsel he'd come for physiotherapy. Upon yet more medical counsel, he'd come to me for swallowing therapy, as it seemed whatever was shaking this man had also invaded the anatomy that ensured his sustenance.

As all diligent inquisitors of my profession do, he wondered aloud why he'd been referred to a speech-language pathologist for a swallowing problem. I acknowledged by way of 'next-door neighbors are the vocal cords—the starters of speech—and the esophagus, transporter of food and drink parcels. Sometimes the delivery worker accidentally brings the esophagus's parcel to the vocal cords, which also happen to be near the lungs' chambers. The vocal cords do not like visitors, you see. Any stranger who comes in potentially brings chaos and ill-health to the sterile chambers the cords maintain. To them, the parcels only harbor the germs of the outside world. One too many "gifts" and their chambers may breed infection and inflammation, which can develop into pneumonia. Because we "speechies" have wonderful knowledge of this neighborhood, we have the honor of ensuring that gifts are routed to the stomach through the esophagus and not to the vocal cords. Thus it is my goal for you not to have food in your airway. I aspire for you to get well, and I aspire for you to aspire to do the same. I do not aspire for you to aspirate. Certainly, aspiration is not our aspiration.'

After I spent a few days working with him, the shaking man told me about his unsettling dreams. Immediately before the first of his tremors, he had dreamed of a man and his four adult sons who had come as strangers from the breeze and set up a debt-collecting firm next to the shaking man's house. They called their business simply Park & Sons.

'Every night, at the darkest minute, they come dressed in white. They invade my house to demand debt be repaid.'

The quivering man, incredulous, always told them that he did not owe money to anyone, that he had paid the last of his debts six years earlier and had the receipt to prove it. Still, Park & Sons invaded night after night, taking a few coins and notes and property. They threatened that they would take all from the man eventually and leave him to waste away.

'I have the dream nearly every night,' said the shaking man, 'and each time, the man and his sons take more from me than they have before.'

Although I am not one for superstition, the steely fear and conviction the man displayed as he related his nightmares compelled me to believe that somehow they were manifesting in his reality. First there had been the case of his weakened muscles warranting physiotherapy, and now the dysphagia—the swallowing difficulty. What next?

As the weeks went on and the man told me of his latest encounters with the malevolent debt collectors, his demeanor changed. Whatever the color of London's sky is in winter, that was the shade of his face. He soon had difficulty centering his body when he walked and shortly after was resigned to a wheelchair. How cruel for an infant to wrestle himself from the pram only to be forced back in as a man. He'd been a spry athlete once, and now his muscles were sore and stiff from the beatings he received from Park & Sons.

Many sessions did we have. Many times did I watch him eat, the shaking man. Many times did the food and drink slip into his airway instead of his stomach, causing him to cough as his nose ran, his clear, crisp voice turned into eddies of gasps. Many times did I ask myself, *Why must we breathe and eat so closely together, with only a thin wall separating these life-sustaining channels, only a fleshy flap protecting life's breath from food?* How cruel that the holy design of homo sapiens must endure such a flaw. I wish the poet Robert Frost's words applied here, for you see, two roads diverge in our red bodies but not quickly enough, not swiftly enough.

Park & Sons continued pillaging. The man continued to owe no debt, but this was of no use. 'And so my body I steel as they still steal,' said the shaking one.

The swallow sessions ticked on. For all his darkness now, the shaking man worked harder in our treatments than any patient before him. We used detailed and technical exercises to protect his airway and improve his swallow. 'Tuck your chin, hold your breath, bear down, swallow hard, swallow again, cough gently, swallow fast, say ahhhhhhhhhh.' Sometimes we needed the aid of technology, of tingling electricity applied to the neck and chin to resurrect Lazarus muscles. Other times we simply used the collective wisdom of mothers past, present and future: 'smaller bites', 'slow down'.

While the debt collectors ransacked at night, we kept working. The long-term plan was to enable my patient to experience as many enjoyable eating sessions as possible and to delay the rate with which Park & Sons caused his swallowing to deteriorate.

When he learned how to effectively stop food from going into his airway, I said he no longer needed my services. By our last session we had arrived at a modified diet; food became softer, meats were chopped up, and he disciplined his fluid intake with small sips and slurps. As we agreed, all of this would allow him to maintain his dignity and the joy of feasting, while it ensured that his throat could safely accommodate his primeval urge to be an alpha omnivore.

Not long after the end of our therapist–patient relationship, I came across the man while on a weekend stroll by the River Thames. Serendipity united us at the Ferris wheel's leaden-eyed reflection in the South Bank. We exchanged hellos and pleasantries. The shaking man had a slight smile on his face, which took me aback as I had grown accustomed to seeing a flat and numb countenance on his best days.

'Strangely enough,' he told me, 'Park & Sons haven't attacked me in a long while. They wait in the shadows of my doorstep, make no mistake, pacing menacingly back and forth ... but that's it, nothing more.'

As I saw his smile broaden and let the breadth of his words sink into my mind's rivers, I freed a breath from my chest's cage. No attacks, only restless pacing, no debts to collect: this, it seemed, was good enough for my once-patient, and on that blue London day it was good enough for me too.

Part II

'Park & Sons' intermission is over,' the shaking man told me when our therapist–patient relationship resumed at my Shoreditch clinic. 'I had another of thosedreamslastnighanatheycamiere ...'

His quivering had increased, joints even stiffer, breathing more labored, movement less fluid. There were dark circles under his eyes and tufts of his hair were gone, his color almost wiped away.

This time he was here because the debt collectors were trying to silence him. They schemed to steal his speech, the very thing he used to recount their assaults or to protest against them or to ask for help. This trick up their sleeve is known as dysarthria: the Greeks and Romans defined it as speech that is disjointed as a result of weak muscles.

Park & Sons wanted to make him incoherent, for no one listens to an incoherent man's words. No one listens to the man whose lips curve in a downward droop even when he isn't sad. No one listens to the man whose exhausted speech muscles will not let him properly utter a dignified 'r' or a distinguished 's' or a delicate 'm'. Who will listen when he speaks but his voice is too quiet? Who will honor his time when his mouth moves but sound does not come? It seems nobody wants to stay around for a re-enactment of Babel where many of the words are difficult to understand.

When the shaking man's words started strong but trailed off—like the metro growing quieter as it leaves me for fair Camden Town—it was much easier for us to talk over him, to cut him off or to finish his sentences.

Minutes after the session ended, I went into the restroom and beheld him in a most vulnerable state. He was leaning in the doorway to a stall, stumbling from the toilet to his wheelchair. His fingers were pale from the grip he had on the stall door.

I asked him, 'Are you all right?' But it was only a courtesy, as the answer was obvious.

He piped up. 'Yes, fine.'

I had always admired the shaking man's tenacity, his determination when all logic deemed his chances unfavorable, when his morning alarm taunted a defeatist, *No, today you cannot achieve anything. You dare not hope against all hope.* Throughout my knowing him, I had often seen him in the corridors taking painful-looking steps as was his ritual after our sessions, determined not to be confined to the wheelchair.

Yet now as his grip loosened and his body lurched towards the ground, he revised his answer to 'no', tears in his eyes. 'I need help, about to fall,' he added, as though admitting defeat.

I placed myself between him and the cold linoleum, but by protocol did not try to catch him, so as to avoid losing my balance and injuring us both. Instead, I gave him a loose embrace from behind, slowly cushioning his descent. As he slid down, I planted one leg and gradually sank into a kneeling posture with one knee touching the ground. There seemed to be a beauty in this gesture; by kneeling and lowering myself, I was symbolically showing solidarity to the man, signifying that he wasn't alone and that people would fall with him if that's what it took to face Park & Sons. It seems in life we paradoxically often take to one knee and lower ourselves in order to be made higher in a firm stance against adversity.

And so the shaking man and I again did battle with Park & Sons. They hatched their plans and made their attacks in the dead of night; we strategized and defended ourselves in broad daylight. It seemed we knew something they didn't: darkness always dies when it touches light.

The shaking man donned his battle gear. At boot camp we disciplined the sober slurring. I led him in drills of tongue twisters: 'pa-ta' turned into 'butter', 'ka' turned into 'cup'—'pa-ta-ka, buh-ta-ka, butter-ka, buttercup', over and over and over and over. In reading and in speaking, precision was our obsession, and so I prescribed a slow rhythm. No need for a polka, just a waltz to synchronize every soldier to achieve clear and crisp annunciation. Lip, jaw, teeth, tongue, throat, uvula, nose: in time, these sergeants came to understand their directive, their war waltz. To make precision excellent, we added the element of overexaggerating the articulators. It was best for him to overemphasize every movement with deliberation and conviction.

But of course there were two sides to this war. Having lost the battle of articulation, Park & Sons found new areas to attack. Each day the shaking man presented himself to camp with his latest battle wounds: the dry mouth, the tremors, the slow movements, the stiffness and the unsteady gait. What unnerved me most was the voice crackles. Park & Sons had learned something we had hoped to keep a secret from them: cut off your enemy's lines of communication and you have the upper hand, as this causes frustration and panic and desperation. And so we fought this angle of attack. Every day the man battled as his voice wavered and at times went silent while his lips and tongue continued their movements for the sounds of his beloved language, his beloved alphabet.

To combat this he learned to have a near-yogic calm. 'Breathe deep into your belly,' I would tell him, 'hold, let it out slowly through parted lips. Roll your head clockwise, slowly, gently. Tense your shoulders upward, and gently relax them downward.' And he learned to be a river: by drinking water often, finishing his cup at least three times a day, he keep his vocal cords hydrated.

Park & Sons took a new approach to slow the battle and the man down to their speed. He was now unsure of many things—of planning actions and using information, and even of his bearings on time and date and place. He now seemed like a train bound on one journey, unable to change course, inflexible. A stupor came over him, and he felt nothing for celebration or alarm, even if he was headed for disaster. At times his train lights would pierce through the fog to reveal a scene in the distance, but it would prove to be a mirage once the train reached that place.

All of a sudden the shaking man would fall asleep, even with sun in the sky. Upon waking, he would apologize. The sweat of his body had developed a habit of leaking, his skin slick with the sheen of oil.

Park & Sons ensured the man's speaking apparatus matched the dulled train lights of his personality. His speech became quiet, a near whisper. Even worse, he could no longer carry a full chorus save for the low flat drone of his one tone, a hymn written for a single note. For this we unleashed officers previously at our base: we summoned the physician and the psychiatrist. To restore the train lights to their former brightness required a whole team. Tirelessly we worked, buffing and shining and tinkering with the bulbs until the lights flooded the world once again with a golden beam. Yet, we didn't stop.

The shaking man strolled with me through the corridors of my clinic, stopping to practice crystalline speech with anyone who would give us half a moment. A dutiful student, he agreed to do homework, to speak to his spouse and friends and acquaintances, not minding so much the what of conversations but more so the how. He must have wanted high marks, as he even went on town outings, speaking to strangers and using their unfamiliarity as a gauge of his progress.

Like that of a master of the theater, his voice filled space, his mouth opened wide and long, and his breath was a gale, the air of which moved through his mouth and nose chambers to amplify his speech. He placed emphasis on all the right words, and his notes moved up at the end of each question. He could make sudden exclamations, while for solemn expressions his sombre notes fluttered downwards.

At the clinic we confirmed this, using a machine that visualized acoustic signals. Months earlier, our graphs recording his speech-air particles had looked like flat plains, at best mounds of earth; now we saw fully formed valleys and mountain tops.

One day after a session, he told me he was a poet and had loved doing readings, but after his diagnosis of dysarthria he had confined himself to writing. 'Now I've survived this round of attacks from Park & Sons, I'm going to do readings again. I've actually signed up for an open mic tomorrow.'

~

Tomorrow came, and I went to the open mic as a listener.

He began: 'I met the therapist in London Town. In a red Tube cab, his eyes were glued to the movements of my hands, ticking, repetitive …' Through every turn of phrase and every pause, I heard his words. I heard them crisply, fully, with each rise and fall of intonation. I heard them loudly—not that he needed much volume, for we the listeners had hushed enough to hear the ghost of a breeze. When he said the last word of his poem, he received one of the loudest rounds of applause and finger snaps of the open-mic hour.

I knew then that Park & Sons would have another hiatus. None the fool, I anticipated there would be more attacks to come—perhaps for the man's brain, the control center itself. However, this win was enough to banish misery for a while. The look on the face of my twice-patient told me he knew what I was thinking, and the smile that followed told me he was content for now and that I needn't worry. This victory was splendid enough for him, and on a green London day it was splendid enough for me too.

Anne

Josie Byrne

My sister Anne had been suffering from depression and I was becoming increasingly worried about her. I would phone her every day from work at 4 p.m. but on this particular day, for some unknown reason, I called at midday.

Me: Hi, Peter, it's Auntie Josie, is your mum there?
Peter: I'll just get her for you—she's in the bathroom.

I heard banging, and Peter's voice.

Peter: Mum, it's Auntie Josie on the phone. Mum? Mum? Answer me!

He came back to the phone.

Peter: She won't answer. She's been in the bathroom for ages.
Me: I'm coming down now.

I dashed out of work, leaving everything, and rang my boss to say I had to go on urgent family business. He was really understanding.

I drove like a madwoman on the country roads. I knew something was wrong, I just knew. There was a tractor in front of me—I tried to overtake it, but that was impossibly dangerous on the twisting, narrow lane.

The voice in my head: You're overreacting, you always do. Why do you panic? Everything's all right, she's just having a long bath. But why did she not answer Peter? Why wouldn't she come and talk to you?

At last the tractor moved off, and I could put my foot down a bit. I arrived at my sister's house and was greeted by Peter.

Me: Has she come out yet?

Peter: No, I told her that you were coming, but she won't speak to me.

I went inside. Everything was the normal, lovely home it had always been. At the bathroom door I knocked.

Me: Hi, Anne, it's Josie.

No reply.

Me: Will you open the door, Anne?

No reply.

Me: Come on, Anne, I've driven from work, please open the door.

Nothing.

Me to Peter: How long has she been in there?
Peter: About an hour.

So long?

Me: Listen, Anne, if you don't come out of there by the time I count to ten, I am going to call the fire brigade to come and break the door down.

No reply.

Me: I'm going to start counting backwards, and if you haven't come out by the time I get to one, I'm calling. Ten … nine … eight …

I was laughing a little at myself now and thinking, *How dramatic are you?* Anne and I would laugh about this later.

Anne: Who's there with you?
Me: Just Peter.
Anne: Tell him to go upstairs.
Me: Peter, go upstairs.

He left.

Me: Four … three … two …

Then she unlocked the door. Nothing in my life, before or since, equipped me for what I saw when the door opened.

The first thing I registered was how white the bath was. Then I realised that was because there was so much blood. My beautiful sister was standing naked, her wrists cut. Blood everywhere, on the walls, floor, all over her pale body.

She just stood there saying, 'Oh, I've done it now. I've really made a mess of things.'

Peter was there, his nineteen-year-old face contorted with horror. It twisted into the face of an old man. He started to cry.

I wanted to protect my nephew, to put my arms around him and tell him that it would be all right, but I had to take care of my sister.

I screamed at her, 'What have you done?! What have you done?!'

She just kept saying, 'I've made a mess of things now, I've made such a mess of things.'

I shouted to Peter, 'Go upstairs and ring your dad.'

I dialled 999.

999: Police, Ambulance, Fire, which do you require?
Me: Ambulance, my sister has cut her wrists.
999: Was it an accident, or did she do it on purpose?
Me: On purpose.
999: Get some towels, wrap them tightly around her wrists. Really tight, do you understand? Someone will be with you shortly.
Me: Okay.

I went to get the towels. I wrapped them around her poor cut wrists. Her eyes had changed, turned cloudy. She was groggy.

Peter came downstairs.

Me: Go upstairs, contact your dad—now!

I wanted to get my sister some clothes.

In the midst of the horror, I heard knocking at the door. A voice said, 'Hello!' It was my frail ninety-year-old dad. I didn't want him to see his daughter naked and like this.

Too late, he was in. The look on his face when he saw his daughter; he started to shake.

'Dad, Dad!' I screamed. 'Go into the other room!' Peter took him to sit down in the lounge.

I heard a wail.

I wanted to find clothes for my sister. I went to her bedroom and found some jogging bottoms and a top. I dressed her. She stood, zombie-like, her eyes misted over. After she was clothed I took her into the kitchen to sit down. There was no expression on her face. She didn't speak. She started to rock, rock, rock. Faster and faster. A rhyme formed in my mind.

Rocking sister with cloudy eyes,
listen to my sighs

How strangely the mind works.

I heard sirens, the ambulance. The twenty minutes it took them seemed like twenty hours.

The ambulance team were fast and efficient. They asked where her medication was, to check if she had taken any. They wrapped a blanket around her. I went with her in the ambulance.

In accident and emergency people stared at us, and I wanted to shout at them, *Look away! Look away!* But they didn't, and we had to sit with everyone else. After about an hour, her name was called and we were taken to a cubicle. No questions were asked. The doctor started to stitch Anne's wrists, and she just sat there, expressionless.

Arthur, Anne's husband, arrived with panic in his eyes. He hugged and kissed her, held her hands and told her he loved her. My sister said nothing.

When we hugged, he said, 'I'm glad that this has happened—they'll have to do something now.'

We sat in A&E from 1 p.m. until 9 p.m., waiting for a psychiatrist who would determine if Anne needed sectioning. Eventually one came. He took Anne into a separate room, and Arthur and I had to wait outside.

The psychiatrist talked with Anne for about half an hour before he called us in. He told us she was extremely ill, that this wasn't a cry for help. He said she would have to be sectioned and would be taken to the Leigh Hospital Psychiatric Unit. One of the things that Anne had told him was that she was responsible for her nephew getting cancer.

I waited with Anne another hour for transport, and I went with her while Arthur followed in his car. Anne still hadn't spoken much. I filled the silence with my own words; I told her that she would be well, that she was going to be safe.

I don't think she heard anything.

At Leigh Hospital, we saw a psychiatrist who asked Arthur and me many questions about Anne and our childhood. I told him what I could about our past, and he wanted to know more. Arthur, so protective, tried to conceal how difficult our childhood had been, but I didn't cover anything up. I wanted Anne to get better, and if this was the path to recovery, however painful it was for me, I would walk it. I told him.

When I left the hospital it was 1 a.m., and I was exhausted. I realised the only thing I'd ingested that day was a cup of coffee. I remembered I had to present at a meeting in the college the next day. That night I didn't sleep but replayed the day's events over and over. In the morning I went to my job in a dream-like state. At times I thought perhaps none of it had happened.

The next day I visited Anne in hospital, where she was in a room on her own. Two senior psychiatrists told me that in all their years of practice, they had never seen anyone as ill as my sister.

She hadn't eaten or washed. She lay on the floor, curled in a ball. She still believed that she'd done something that made her undeserving of a bed or food. My sister was a gentle person; she'd helped so many people during her life. She wouldn't speak or look at me. She kept saying, 'When you find out what I have done, you'll never speak to me again.' She had, of course, done nothing.

~

Two weeks later she was no different. I visited her every evening to try to get her to shower and eat, with no success. She was so thin and dulled after weeks of not eating or bathing. After hours of bargaining, I persuaded her to go out for a walk with me. But only five minutes later she collapsed, and I shouted for a nurse.

Anne was on a lot of drugs, but they weren't effective, so the doctors told us that they were going to try electroconvulsive therapy. Arthur and I were initially taken aback, but then it seemed the only option as she was going so rapidly downhill. The ECT was scheduled for the following day.

The evening after the ECT, I wasn't permitted to visit, but I went the day after. Surprisingly, my sister was so much better. She was calmer, talked more and made eye contact.

Anne had three more ECT sessions and improved after each one. I was filled with something that resembled hope.

After two months, we were allowed to take her home for a long weekend. Arthur picked her up and planned for a quiet time at home. Anne slept a lot. Nothing was specifically wrong, but something felt not right to me.

She was upset on the Monday when she had to go back to the unit.

After ten weeks, the doctors said she could come home. She'd started eating normally, was talking more and had regained weight. I found out much later that one of the doctors had told Arthur to tie her to the bedpost, to prevent her from self-harming again. Arthur tried to find a balance between letting her have her own space, and that warning.

Anne phoned me when she got home. We had long conversations, and I felt like I had her back.

~

Bang, bang on my front door. It was 1 a.m. but I wasn't asleep yet. I went downstairs. I saw the shapes of two people through the front-door glass.

When I opened the door, the people were revealed as police officers. They asked me to confirm my name. After that the world stopped. 'Who is it?' I asked.

One of the officers said that it was my sister, that she had hung herself.

For a brief sickening moment I felt relief that it wasn't about my son.

The phone rang. I sank to the floor, understanding my life had changed forever.

On the phone was Arthur's brother, warning me that the police were on their way.

My husband and I drove to Arthur's house; there were police cars everywhere. When I walked the garden path, I heard what I thought was an animal in a trap. Then I realised it was Arthur, wailing.

He told us later that they'd had a beautiful day. They'd been for a walk and spoken about going on holiday somewhere warm, after Christmas. When they came home, Anne tidied up and made a steak-and-kidney pie, Arthur's favourite. In the evening she convinced him to go to the local pub for a drink, which had been one of his favourite habits, before. After much persuasion, he went. He was only gone for an hour. When he returned and opened the front door, a terrible sight greeted him.

Lifelines

Annette Freeman

My thoughts were perfectly lucid, neatly parsed and clearly enunciated. But only a strange croak sounded in the hospital room: 'Help me.'

These words hadn't been in my mind at all. In my mind I was giving the medical staff information, things it might be useful for them to know: *I don't feel any pain. There was a lot of blood; it's in the bathroom. Have a look, see what you think. I'm having trouble moving my arms.*

But all I said, faintly, was, 'Help me.'

When the croak came out, the two interns on either side of the bed stopped for a moment and glanced at my face. Nurses were in the room too; I couldn't tell how many. Someone was busy at my wrist, inserting something. No one answered me. They seemed surprised that I had spoken at all. I couldn't lift my head or my arms; my lips had barely moved, and after croaking out the two words I said nothing else.

It must have been about three or four in the morning, I worked out later. The baby had been born at 1.13 a.m. That time had been carefully recorded. It was a boy, my third baby. The birth had been quick but not easy. He was big, facing the wrong way, and delivered with a clanking machine called a vacuum extractor. He was *extracted* rather than birthed. We hugged him, his father and I, and shared a cup of tea in the dark small hours in the quiet hospital. Then he was taken to the nursery, and his father went home to sleep.

The night-shift nurse took me, the new mother, in a wheelchair to the bathroom. She left me to shower, and I watched blood swirling down the drain. It looked like a lot of blood; only I saw it.

When the nurse returned she brought a dry hospital gown, helped me slip my arms into it and position a fat pad between my legs.

'There was a lot of blood,' I told her.

'Oh, that's just normal,' she said. Then she helped me into the wheelchair and pushed me through the quiet corridors to the admissions desk. I was being transferred from the delivery suite to the maternity ward; I suppose there was admin to do.

One nurse said to the other, 'She thinks she's lost a lot of blood, but it's all normal.' Her tone was cheerful. *Perhaps delivering babies is a happy job*, I thought.

I was taken to a private room and helped into the hospital bed. I felt tired, as you can imagine. Though I wasn't really comfortable, I dozed. My breasts filled with milk, and my uterus oozed blood. My legs were tired. My head and heart were full. I had a baby. All my thoughts zeroed in on both the baby and my body.

I felt the pad between my legs become saturated with blood. It woke me, and I climbed out of bed and went into the bathroom where there was a toilet. Blood ran down my legs. Cleaning up was awkward. As I swabbed at the blood with toilet paper, more and more ran out. Blood made the toilet bowl red and soon covered the bathroom floor. I wiped and swabbed, but it was beyond me. It occurred to me again that this was too much, though I remembered hearing somewhere that if you spilled just half a cup of blood, it would look like a lot more. The nurse would know for sure, I thought.

I decided to leave the bathroom as it was, to show her. She hadn't believed me when the blood had washed down the shower drain; she hadn't been able to see it. So I staunched the flow with a fresh pad, left the bathroom as it was and climbed back into bed, onto sheets already smeared with maroon. It was silent in the middle of the night. The room smelled reassuringly of hospital disinfectant and ironed linen.

I slept again; I woke again. I felt the pad full again, the bed wet around me. I lifted my fingers, and they came up bloody. I was lying in a pool of it. How curious to sense the body exsanguinate, without pain. Just emptying, like a jug of water with a crack in it. I thought, *I must call the nurse to help me change this sheet. It's too wet. I must press the call button and get help with this.* I knew the button was on the high bedside table. It was emergency red, set in a grey housing and connected by a cord to something in the wall.

'Just press it if you need me,' the nurse had said.

My mind was clear on the action needed: lean the right arm across, take the button in the hand, press it. Some time passed while I turned this thought over. I moved my head so I could see the button. Had I pressed it? I drifted into an uncanny place where time acted strangely, standing still and speeding up simultaneously. It seemed ages before the nurse arrived, before the room filled with people, before they wheeled in a stand with a drip, before they were all talking over me with indistinct words.

On the other hand, the things that happened next also seemed to happen in a great rush. The nurse strode in and greeted me cheerfully, wrapped a blood-pressure sleeve around my arm and read the result. She dropped the pressure bulb with a clash on the table and ran from the room. Her footsteps skittered down the corridor. At first I was mildly amused because she was running indoors. Then it dawned on me that running probably indicated something bad. But I felt no pain, no distress. I drifted.

More hurrying feet sounded. Several men came in, not in white coats but in shirts and with stethoscopes. They held my wrists; they checked my blood pressure again. A nurse, possibly the same one, pushed the drip stand into the room; it clattered. Someone shoved something hurriedly into the back of my right wrist (there was a bruise later) and hung a bag of clear fluid above me on the drip stand. In my head I conveyed my helpful information, joining the conversation.

Out of my mouth came only the involuntary words: 'Help me.'

They glanced at me as if I'd spoken from a faraway place.

Later I learned that the blood pressure reading had been profoundly low, and I'd shown symptoms of going into something called hypovolemic shock. I'd never paid much attention to blood pressure before, just vaguely supposed that it measured the pressure of the blood as it moved through veins. My body at that moment had much less blood to pump. That morning I was given six units of plasma and four units of whole blood. There was a delay in getting the blood as they had to double-check my blood type and find a supply. Donated by someone with blood to spare, I supposed.

~

It was midmorning when I woke again, in an operating theatre. A nurse stood near my shoulder, and I asked for my baby. I started to cry. To my relief, they brought the baby, handed him into the crook of my arm. I fed him a little and eased my bloated breasts. I stared into his newborn eyes, concentrated on feeding him, forgot the stricken night. Then he was whisked away. Gone.

The doctor came—the specialist, the one who'd delivered the baby. He seemed pissed off. They hauled my legs into stirrups, and he poked about, swabbing off blood, trying to see the source of the problem like a mechanic under the hood of a car. At about this point I found the anaesthetic I'd been given for the birth, for the *extraction*, had worn off. Every time the doctor touched me, I flinched.

He became more pissed off. Eventually he took off his white coat and flung it on the floor in a temper, a nurse scurrying to pick it up. He told me that since I wouldn't submit to him touching me, I'd need to have a general anaesthetic, which would be bad for the baby, and for feeding. I lay on the examination table, mortified. Of course I wanted to do the best thing for my baby. But my flinches from the doctor's painful touch were automatic. His scolding made me feel like a child, not a mother.

An anaesthetist arrived. He told me I would only need a light anaesthetic and that the procedure shouldn't take long. He covered my mouth and nose with a mask, and I drifted. The strange state lasted a long time and was filled with vivid dreams, to do with numbers and the solving of complex arithmetical problems. I woke. The doctor and the anaesthetist were still beside me, talking. They were talking numbers.

They looked at me, and one said, 'She's awake.'

I learned later that it'd taken the doctor two hours to repair, with tiny internal stitches, the damage done to my uterus and cervix by the birth, the *extraction*. At his first visit to my bedside afterwards the doctor told me I'd be fine. At his next visit he said it was lucky the baby was a boy, because now I had two girls and one boy and wouldn't want any more children. At his final visit he said it was not recommended that I ever have another pregnancy.

The baby seemed to thrive. The evening after he was born, while feeding him again, I heard an announcement on a television. Somewhere in the USSR, in a place called Chernobyl, a nuclear reactor had exploded. There were fearful predictions of creeping radiation shrouding Europe, of mass destruction, the possible end of the world. I scoffed. Didn't I have new life in my arms, less than a day old? It wasn't possible that living wouldn't go on, full of promise.

My son's birthday through the years would be flagged by anniversary stories of the meltdown. His fifth birthday, his tenth, his twenty-fifth, linked forever to Chernobyl. A birthday and a deathday.

~

Some years later I sat at a small table covered with a velvet cloth, faded purple. There was an aroma of cheap incense. The fortune-teller had set out the cloth, the incense and a candle to create an atmosphere of mystical possibility. She had a corner, behind a curtain, in a New Age bookshop. She didn't wear a headscarf or gold earring, but they were implied. My right hand was in hers, palm up. She peered closely at it, then announced I would have only three children (correct) and would be married once (who could tell?).

Then she gave a dramatic gasp. 'Your lifeline!' she said. 'Something happened when you were about thirty. What was it?'

'No … no,' I said, 'nothing life-threatening has happened to me, nothing at all.'

She insisted. 'There's a clear break in the lifeline, a clear break. It's in your hand. It's so.'

I left the shop. It'd been amusing to have my fortune read. I looked at my right palm: the lines did form a strange Y-shaped pattern. Had my life really cracked, almost off course, when I was thirty? It was only then, after I'd left the fortune-teller, that I remembered.

Unlearning

Sarah Sasson

What do you call the evening if it's not dark? It was midsummer and 9 p.m. The sky still held light in a way I wasn't used to and I couldn't unwind until the clouds released it. I'd tried to explain this to colleagues at the John Radcliffe Hospital. 'In Sydney we only really have two seasons: hot and sunny and less hot, still sunny.'

I appreciated the getting to here—the Thames Valley's turning of the seasons. Autumn, when the leaves became golden and really did fall. Spring, when the bald skeletons of trees exploded with coloured petals. Small armies of daffodils erected where once there had been only grass. The months here marked time in a heavy-handed way, forced us to appreciate what of it we had.

In the depths of winter my husband and I slept longer and longer; in the morning I had to rub the backs of our children to wake them. An incomplete hibernation. I'd never noticed before, how programmed humans are by the sun; how we rise and fall with light, like sea monkeys.

But summer created its own challenge. I didn't feel tired until midnight, then before 5 a.m. the sun cut through the room like a blade; some nights I only clocked four hours of sleep. We bought thick blackout blinds from the hardware store and installed them ourselves. Every time I lowered them I thought of Al Pacino in *Insomnia*, taping the edges of his blinds to Alaskan windows in the small town of Nightmute. In the film it's summer, and Pacino is an out-of-town detective unable to sleep in 24-hour light. Robin Williams played the villain in that movie.

I grew up watching *Mork & Mindy* after school on the wicker couch of our sunroom. Williams's Mork stood outside his egg-shaped spaceship in bright colours, speech racing, effervescent. I found it hard to reconcile Mork being performed by the same actor as the sinister, hermetic Nightmute writer. The transformation seemed to personify how insomnia could leech colour, turn sitcom into noir.

I knew the syrupy nausea of long days on no sleep, the heart-race of overtiredness. I pulled the blinds down to their limit.

I wasn't going back.

~

The birth of my second child, my daughter, was not like that of my older son. My first labour broke my body open in new faultlines. With A—, it was as if I walked down an already trodden path. She was born into the world rounded, pink and screaming: a noisy peach.

The problems started later, after the flowers and gifts subsided, the onset insidious in the hours of the night. Rising to feed the baby, rising to comfort the toddler. With my husband away with work, there was much rising and falling. My children were a garden that needed tending to around the clock. Time began to lose meaning. The number no longer mattered, only what needed to be done.

One night I lay in bed wide awake, and it felt counterproductive to try and fall asleep. Better to stay alert for the next cycle of comforting, rather than be jolted from sleep, feeling groggy.

~

When I was a junior doctor I worked hospital night shifts. For a week at a time I'd arrive at 10.30 p.m. for handover, then spend the night reviewing patients and re-charting medications, fluids and analgesia. I wore a small black pager clipped at the waist, and when it beeped the screen lit up green with the ward I was required on. Sometimes I had to run. Once I climbed on a bed to give CPR.

Once I had to assess someone's neurological observations in the early hours. A nurse handed me an oversized yellow flashlight, like the ones used when people had to go into mines, or a forest. When I approached the patient he was asleep. The beam of my light hit his face, and before I knew what was happening he'd woken and swung his arm out to punch me in the head. To this day I'm unsure how I managed to dodge it.

There's no elation like the feeling of finishing a week of night shifts. To crawl between clean sheets for that first sleep afterwards, knowing the pager has been handed off and is someone else's responsibility. Breakfast tastes better, the shower feels hotter, the sky looks more beautiful at the edges.

During my last term as a junior doctor I went up to the roof terrace of the hospital. I took a photo of the dawn breaking over the beach-side suburb. *Sunrise after my last set of night shifts. Ever*, I captioned it on Instagram.

Being a new parent is a bit like doing night shifts after the day shifts, only it doesn't end after a week.

~

'I'm so tired,' I told my friend who also had children.

'Oh, I know.'

I tried to tell people how I felt, but somehow it was interpreted as the punchline to a joke, or a motion of camaraderie.

'I'm exhausted.'

'Me too.' I was so fatigued I was coming apart at the seams, but in a way strangely undiscernible to other people. It was as though I was speaking into a deep well.

Sleep was my Achilles heel, my Sampson's hair; a lack of it, over time, formed kryptonite. My need for rest was all I could think about; without it I couldn't function. I hungered for it.

'I'm *physiologically* tired,' I tried.

The words travelled down, and in the end I was their only listener; they returned to me with centres slightly loosened.

~

In the 2010 film *Inception*, Leonardo DiCaprio, Elliot Page and their team travel through sleep to embed thoughts in people's subconscious minds. There are dreams within dreams within dreams, like matryoshka dolls. The first layer, a rainy Los Angeles sidewalk; the second, a hotel; the third, a fortress on a snow-covered mountain.

I couldn't get to the place where dreams happened. My mind

whirred. I scratched at the surface of sleep, as if the conscious world imprisoned me. I clawed until my nails broke off at the quick; still I couldn't get past the first myoclonic jerk.

'Nothing's as lonely as not sleeping,' Williams taunts Pacino down the phone line.

My problem was not of initiating sleep but of being frequently woken: to feed my daughter, or change my son's wet sheets. I was left only gliding across the surface of slumber, like an ice skater, when I needed to fall through into cold blue depths. I was separated from the abstract layers of rapid eye movement, where ideas are filed, fragments of stories are put together in new ways, and the mind downloads information and reboots itself. I needed to reach the rhythmic eye-shifting cocoon, that nightly restorative baptism.

~

The strangest revelation of a second child is also the same thing everyone warns you about—that she would not simply resemble my first. My son, from an early age, dozed with little effort and in various locations. I'd discovered this when I once left him awake and surrounded by pillows on the floor as I moved into the kitchen to wash up dishes, and when I returned his small arms were stretched above his head; he was supine and slumbering, a bather in the sun.

In contrast, from the moment my daughter was on the outside she had a strong and animalistic need to be close to me. Following birth she rooted herself to my left nipple and began sucking. She sucked so relentlessly, my milk supply came in a day early. In order to sleep, she needed to be held. I'd never planned on co-sleeping but often found her in my arms midmorning, nodding off, me in submission.

When A— was a bit older, she did a strange, primal thing. As I held her, she turned her face into my bare forearm and ran her tongue and gums up and down my skin until it was wet with her saliva. Then she pressed her cheek into me over the wetness.

I looked in parenting books but couldn't find an explanation for what she was doing.

I showed it to my mother, who watched quizzically, then squinted and said, 'It's as if she's sealing herself onto you.'

A— wrote on me in saliva using a toothless ridge, but the message was clear: *I need you in ways that are both ancient and new.*

I lifted my arm to smell it, expecting to detect whatever magical soothe-scent I emitted. It was as if she inhaled a kind of particulate anxiolytic. But when I put my nose to my forearm it was neutral, or sometimes held the faint smell of our soap.

~

When A— was three months old, my husband travelled overseas for work. The night he left I stayed up and browsed Netflix. There was something calming about scrolling through a bottomless list of movies that was cultivated, apparently, for me. Critically acclaimed. Indie/Arthouse. Films with a strong female lead. I felt comforted by the viewing suggestions, as if they'd been offered by a friend—even though I knew it was an algorithm. I selected a movie about a group of young workers who travelled across the American Midwest selling magazine subscriptions. It was nearly 2 a.m. but I didn't feel tired.

I found a bottle of melatonin in the bathroom cupboard; my husband used them after long-hall flights. The label on the back of the bottle said they could be safely used as a sleep aid and should be taken half an hour before bedtime. The top of the jar still had cotton wool inside. I removed it and looked at the white tablets nestled in the jar. I shook out a large tablet, which smelled innocuous. I decided to take one.

On the screen, the magazine-sellers had taken over a supermarket; they were dancing in the checkout lines to a song about finding love in a place without hope.

Once I'd swallowed the tablet, I wondered if there were any negative side effects. When I googled 'melatonin and side effects', I found it shouldn't be used by people who show signs of depression. I'd read so much about postnatal depression at university, online and in pregnancy books. Everyone was primed for it, to be aware in case it happened. Could you get postnatal depression more than three months postpartum?

I googled 'depression'. A common symptom: tiredness. But I felt more distressed than depressed. *Had a mother ever died from lack of sleep?*

I didn't want to risk things. I put my middle finger down the back of my throat and brought up the soft mound of tablet that fizzed with bubbles around its edge. It stuck to the side of the basin like tea-leaves, and when I looked at it I realised that not only did I not know what was wrong with me, but that I'd lost any kind of diagnostic perspective.

In medical school they drummed into us the importance of having our own GP. *Sure*, I thought, *for pap smears and vaccinations.* I was young and well and studying medicine; the reality of needing anything more than cursory care—of being on the other side of the examination—seemed far away.

~

That morning I had an appointment with my GP, Dr Padmanabhan. I attempted to make a bowl of cereal and a cup of tea; I poured boiling water over the Special K and cold milk straight onto my tea bag. I was unsteady on my feet, as if the floorboards were floating logs. I drove down the road with my daughter all bright-faced in her car seat. I thought I had right of way in the roundabout, but the fact that two drivers blasted their horns at me while one nearly ran into us made me unsure.

'My daughter only sleeps for forty minutes twice a day,' I told Dr Padmanabhan, when I was sitting in a beige chair across from her. 'There's no chance to catch up.'

A— leaned in to the doctor from where she sat on my lap and smiled.

'She looks absolutely perfect, and very well cared for,' said Dr Padmanabhan.

That was the issue: the intensity with which she needed me was draining.

'But you can't go on like this, not sleeping,' the doctor said. 'Otherwise, you'll be crushed.'

Midnight on the sixth night was when Pacino snapped; my daughter was three months old.

I watched the doctor as she typed at her computer. I couldn't see the text from where I was sitting. *How strange to be the fixee, rather than the fixer.* Dr Padmanabhan was the first one to see it, the large translucent boulder made up of all the sleep I hadn't had, hanging precariously over me. She printed out a prescription for a higher-dose melatonin than I had at home, one that was sustained release. 'And if you find that's not working, I'll give you something stronger.'

I watched the small machine behind her that spat out printed prescriptions onto green paper, and I felt grateful.

The following night I took the melatonin for the second time and lay in the bath. I had a strange sensation, as if my body was a metal coil relaxing. I realised I hadn't experienced that transition from day to night in a long while—my diurnal rhythm, the slow relaxation of the body preparing to sleep.

~

My son, now three, came home from day care with a report card about what skills he'd mastered and how he interacted with other children. *Was it normal for a child to receive a report card in day care?*

One line stuck with me: 'B— knows how to ask for compassion when he requires it.'

The report went on to describe how he would raise his arms towards his most trusted carer, asking to be lifted and held if needed. It made me wonder if I'd ever gained this milestone, and—if I had—when in adulthood I'd unlearned it.

~

'Cuddle, Mama?'

A— has found me in the kitchen. I hoist her up, and she wraps her arms and legs around me, resting her head on my shoulder. She still needs me in frequent, visceral ways that her older brother never has. Her attachment to me is at the bottom of her hierarchy, the base of her pyramid; I'm her touchstone, rabbit's foot and rosary.

She needs me perhaps in the same way I need sleep. Now that she requires me at times that don't wake me, it has made an overwhelming difference.

When she hangs from me like this, with her rump over my abdomen, I am reminded of when I knew her only from within. I circle my fingers down and around the length of her spine and imagine what shapes they would make if their tips were dipped in ink, a type of calligraphy. I try to decipher the message I am leaving on her back. *I'm here for you: for things that are small, and not small.*

This feels like a continuation of a text, one that will be passed between her and me over many years; we write into each other without an alphabet, and in marks that are not always or entirely seen by eye.

Purgatory

Isabella Mori

The gates of hell are open night and day;
Smooth the descent, and easy is the way:
But to return, and view the cheerful skies,
In this the task and mighty labor lies.

Virgil, *Aeneid*, Book 6

Like those of many older institutions in this city, the buildings of St. Mary's Hospital were mishmashed together: an annex here, a tunnel there, a bridge, a wing, a stair, a ramp. None matched, not quite. Over decades the hospital had turned into a warren, a purgatory of confusion. Third floors had become second; numbers were odd on one side, even on the other, but not everywhere—in Building 3H, room numbers jumped from three to eight for no apparent reason. On one of those between-floors—between the basement and the ground level—was EPT: Emergency Psychiatry Treatment.

In 1968 a young, ambitious doctor of psychiatry had enough verve and, more importantly, moneyed connections, to wrest the fate of psychiatric patients away from doctors obsessed with fixing broken bones and reattaching retinas. He built people with unhappy minds their own sanctuary. The only hitch: the donors freely gave money but showed no interest in aesthetics, nor indeed in location. So EPT got stuck *somewhere*—an in-between with hardly any light.

In 1981 the young, ambitious doctor had long gone off to Harvard or the Mayo Clinic or wherever young, ambitious doctors went. A kind administrator had found a little money, bought chairs cushioned in cheery orange, painted all the counters green, and retrieved some art from a small gallery gone broke.

Nothing had changed since then. In 2015 EPT was a dark

place, a place of healing and of suffering. One quarter sanctuary, two quarters purgatory, one part a mystery.

Hans was a man of undetermined age (well—no: determined by some scribbles on a chart, immediately forgotten). He came in, hand broken, bloody with glass from the window he had jumped through. The window and the void beyond? Who knew? Clearly to him, at that moment, and with those voices in his mind, jumping had been the thing to do. The police were driving by, heard splintering noises, stopped, and found the shivering man curled on the ground, bloodied but mostly whole.

His third day at the EPT, Hans resumed the medication that had seemed the source of all the evil in his life not long ago. Behind a screen, days one and two: a fog of needles, doctors in suits, security guards, nightmares, a padded, dark room too hot to breathe in. Wrestling. He couldn't remember who or what—his demons? Hospital staff? Another patient? Would not have been the first time.

But now, he liked his nurse. He slept quite well. This came about, he felt, from knowing someone was there, someone who cared, someone who kept him safe. He took willingly what was given to him. Too tired of questioning, of suspecting, and the pills helped him suspect much less. The voices were still by his side, but they murmured more and screamed less often. They spoke more now in what Hans had read somewhere was called 'word salad'. Arugula. Cucumber. 'matos. Matchmakers making egg salad. Less of the 'die!' variety, the voice that hungered for that sound of splintering, of crashing, of crunching bones and wet, dead splattering. Instead, a little bit of mumbled word salad—romaine, abstain, contain—was fine with him.

He watched the others as they picked fights, played cards, screamed, hugged each other. They swore at nurses, wrote them adoring notes, did not accept their doctors' orders.

Hans watched as Jill cried. Jill who couldn't stop the memories of little ones unborn—three little ones—and whose mother came daily in vain hopes of consoling her. Jill's husband was long gone to find another woman, one who would give attention just to him, cheer him up, one who would not forget to put on make-up every day, and pretty shoes.

Hans watched Norm, who wouldn't speak, and Peter, who didn't seem upset at anyone or anything, a guy friendly enough to nurses and to doctors as long as they engaged in endless small talk with him.

'Nice weather, Nurse.'

'Hm.'

'Nice weather, I said, Nurse.'

'Nice weather, Peter.'

Peter staked out meaningless nothings around him. Beyond that, he shared not a bit. He slept and sat, waited in limbo until they found a place for him to stay where he wouldn't break everything he found—chairs, sofas, tables—into pieces. Not that he was angry; it's just he needed someone to talk to. And it wasn't fair when people didn't make time for him. Not fair.

There was Clara, admitted for the first time, and what could be her last. Perhaps she just needed time away, a few nights' sleep, some medication. There were quite a few like her. A rock came smashing through their hearts and minds, the shock horrible, they picked the rock up, threw it back or buried it, and that was it. Maybe they found a way to glaze their windows with thicker glass, maybe they were fortunate and a rock never again came hurtling through.

Many a rock had come through Hans's windows. Many a window had been broken, both from within and without. It had started when his mother jumped, and hadn't ended since. They'd taken his boy away. 'Too dangerous,' they'd said, after his wife had found him, twenty-one years ago, standing on the balcony, holding their child. Unwilling to come in, to move away from the abyss up on the nineteenth floor.

Hans wanted to heal.

~

One nurse, Gretchen, arrived early for each shift at EPT, her limbs heavy, voice tired, skin dried out from smoke and sorrow. She'd seen it all. People who'd attempted suicide came in and then left a day later, and were dead the next. Furious husbands, sleep-deprived brothers, naive girls came to the hospital equipped with vials full of coke, hidden in places who-knew-where. Social workers who didn't give a shit; doctors who didn't think they were God, they *knew* it. Nurses who gossiped, lazed about then snarled at patients.

At one time there had seemed to be more hope, but that was years ago. Or aeons.

Gretchen was suffering. She couldn't hear when Jack, the junior nurse, spoke of a woman with depression whose face lit up when he sat down and listened to her speak about her three cats. She didn't feel Hans's friendly eyes on her. Wouldn't read the book the psychiatrist had lent her about mountains that Sib knew Gretchen once loved very much.

Her heart was blind.

~

Hans dreamt. It woke him up. He found Nurse Gretchen tired and wanting to be alone. She was crocheting—pink, black, beige—behind the desk. But Hans insisted. Gretchen rose, thought about charging him with obstreperousness, even *aggression* (a word highlighted in purple on the chart, a word that was not easily erased), when something stopped her.

'I dreamt,' Hans said, 'of a strange place, in Italy. There was a cave. There was a woman, and she looked like Sibyl, the psychiatrist.'

Gretchen flinched, thinking of Sib's quietness. She didn't like when Sib finally dispensed words—not many—and said things that made her shiver. She didn't like her voice, it made her think of—no. Memories were useless.

Hans went on. 'This old woman looked like your mother. In the dream. I mean, I don't know your mother. But there in Italy I knew her. In my dream there, I knew your mother. She looked a bit like you, just older. Softer, maybe?'

Gretchen took Hans's chart and wrote: *Dreams. Ideas of reference.* Her hand shook. She changed pens. 'That's interesting,' she mumbled.

'Her hair was longer than yours, wavier, and she wore skirts. Another thing I knew about her, don't ask why—this woman didn't like the feel of pants.'

Their eyes, Hans's and Gretchen's, were drawn to Gretchen's gray-blue slacks that she wore every day. They were so practical.

'Well, thank you, Hans,' she said. 'And now it's off to bed with you. Need pills?' He looked at her, wanting to continue. Gretchen turned from him. There were things to do, tasks far away from women who didn't like the feel of pants.

Hans raised a hand and cleared his throat. 'Si—'

'Now, now,' said Gretchen, remembering vaguely what it was like to smile, a real smile.

Hans stopped. Something in him knew about the drums we carry deep inside us, how much it hurts when outside voices make their old hides thrum. He'd received so many good things in this hospital; no need to push it. He went to bed. His face relaxed, a friendly light dancing in his green eyes. And off he went, to dream again.

~

The next day Hans was discharged, just before lunch. He collected what few things he had and walked down the hall. He was free. On the other side of the heavy door he'd been locked behind, someone opened it for him. He had a dim sense that it was spring, the twenty-fifth of May. Disorientation set in. *Where to?* A bare corridor stretched before him: grey to the left, grey to the right. A light bulb flickered; another had gone out completely. Far down on the right was an empty stretcher. He walked along that side of the corridor. His sneakers squeaked on the waxed floor. He smelled nothing, tasted nothing.

He arrived at the stretcher. Three books lay there. He looked around and heard his father's cold voice: *Got nothing to do with you, boy, go, move on!* His father was a harsh, strict man. Malicious, even. Rebelliously, Hans did not heed the voice. His dad's advice was always expensive to his soul. He took the books.

Further ahead he faced three more choices: keep going on, go left, or go halfway to the right. His head reeled. He wanted to return to the safety of the EPT. But there was no way to find the path back. There was nothing left but to go forward.

And then: another human being! A woman in heels. Would she be friendly, helpful?

Hans slowed, hesitation in his steps. His mouth felt dry. 'Excuse me?' he said.

She spoke mostly in Italian and knew little English. She was a Jehovah's Witness, which he found out immediately, and pointed towards what might have been the way out before smiling and handing him three *Watchtower* magazines. Hans heard his father's voice again: *Don't take a thing from these cult idiots! Imbeciles all!*

Polite nevertheless, Hans took the magazines and smiled back. 'Ciao!' He remembered that word from a trip that happened a long time ago. Saying it aloud ignited a small joyous feeling in his chest.

Don't take a thing from these cult idiots! He hadn't obeyed the voice. What's more, he knew it was his father's. A voice not from the outside but from the inside. A voice knitted from memories. He knew now that he could react the way *he* chose. He knew that the voice must obey *him*, and not the other way around.

He looked down at the magazines. It was unlikely he'd read them, but they gave him something that made him feel grateful.

He walked deeper into the labyrinth. He saw pipes above him, and doors with the words *Keep Out! Hazardous Waste! Boiler Room.* He hadn't had lunch yet; his blood sugar felt low. He sat beside *HVAC 2*, down on the floor.

Small. Hans felt small. He said the words aloud. 'Small. I feel very small.' He said this with his own voice; no one else commanded him. Something inside him liked the words. They spoke a truth. The truth was good. 'I feel so small.' He repeated it, tasting the words. What to do now? He did not know. 'I feel small. I do not know.' Hans laughed, a small, content laugh. These truths, they felt so comfortable.

He was sitting beside the door to those who controlled all the weather in this vast old place. Heat, ventilation, air conditioning. Hot, cold, it was up to them. Hans controlled nothing.

He leafed through one found book, then another, *The Anatomy of Peace*. The third was a small, dog-eared paperback copy of Virgil's *Aeneid*, Latin on one side and English on the other. He didn't feel guilty for taking the books. They seemed meant for him. The first had its cover missing. He shook it. Something fell out: three bits of paper. A recipe for brownies, and one for soup. The third was a doodle. *This way out!* a sign read on it, with stars and smiley faces that pointed to an open mouth with flowers sprouting to one side.

Hans looked up. Stood. Picked willy-nilly one of the three branches of the labyrinth that ended in a door. He walked out.

It was spring. May twenty-fifth. The sun shone on a bench in a garden with blooming peonies. Not far off, gleaming beneath blue skies, was a street sign: *9th Avenue.*

Hans nodded, smiled and walked on.

Dive

Sophie Overett

After the appointment, Alice takes her to the beach.

She hadn't meant to, hadn't planned it or promised it, but the doctor had shaken his head and Alice had taken the wrong turn-off, and now they're here, letting the autumnal winds try to set sail with them, their bare toes locked like anchors in sea-spattered sand.

She's never noticed before how many mangroves take up this corner of the beach, their bodies yawning out of seabeds. Fat-bellied gulls with silver crests clutch to their stubborn branches, turning beady black eyes to the water. She can't see it from here, but she knows there are small yellowing guppies and wriggling sandworms beneath the lag of ocean, and it won't be long before the gulls find them, jerking them out with the spears of their beaks.

When Alice was small, smaller anyway, they would spread out here, make sand angels with their narrow bodies, crafting impressions of themselves in the shore until the water soaked in and distorted them—made their impressions these half things and then nothings, like they'd never lain there at all. Kept their secrets, like they've kept this one.

She bites the inside of her cheek, feels the tremble at her bones, from the hard top of her skull to the fine ones of her toes. They never should've come here. She should've taken her home, back to bed, to Alice's already grieving father and the heavy, ancient cat that her mother can't seem to sleep without anymore.

Fisting her car keys, Alice traces the jagged line of them with her fingers, hard enough to break her skin. It doesn't, but the waves do, crashing at their ankles. Alice gasps, her body surging back at the cold of it. Her mother only hisses.

It was the chemotherapy and then the radiation, almost worse than the cancer, that pulled her apart and put her mother back together this way. Fractured and broken. Slimy and strange as a snail with its shell crushed. Her hair and her eyelashes and the downy softness of her that Alice would cling to as a girl were suddenly gone. She's all angles and loose skin now, broken down to sharpness and sag, a coil of desperate, awful parts.

Alice lets out a breath, forces her hands out of their fists and finds that her nails have left half-moon crescents to bleed at her palms. The water breaks at her legs again, hard as a slap, and that's all it takes for her to reach down, jerk at the mouth of her jeans and shove them off. She flings them back towards dryer sand.

Tugging off her t-shirt, she repeats the motion, letting the howling wind catch at the cotton of it and then at her own skin, peaking through the lace of her bra, the elastic of her underwear. The gulls are circling now, calling, and they hesitate to break the frigid water, but Alice doesn't. She runs full bodied into the surf, the water breaking against her bones. Shells and mangrove shoots cut her flesh, but she beats her feet across them anyway, runs in surging steps and thrown-back bounds, depending on the ocean lap. She runs until the sea floor opens up below her like a trap and she has to swim to stay afloat.

Her eyes are stinging, burning from where the salt is trying to shift below her lids. Her legs are aching from the run. Her feet are bleeding.

But it feels good, this burn, this ache, suddenly with cause and reason, a distraction from the swollen one inside her belly, her chest, drowning her dumb, breaking heart. *Please*, she thinks, and she's not sure to who or what for. She wonders if it matters.

A hand at her leg. Another body hogging the cold, deep sea beside her.

And it's her mother, all cellophane skin and eyes bright as broken glass catching shards of light. 'Alice,' her mother says, treading water, her frail body bobbing with every shrug of the sea.

And it's not fair, none of this is fair, least of all her disappearing mother. They were supposed to grow old not together but in tandem, in that round dance a mother and daughter should do, orbiting the same steps, years apart but somehow still together. Like an echo or a ripple. Alice doesn't want this step, doesn't want this transition. Wants to cut out this part of the dance and forget it.

But she can't, so she laughs instead, her mouth filling with water, then her nose, her body sinking as she wishes the gulls would fish her out. But it's her mother who pulls her back to the water's surface, and Alice laughs louder still.

Call of the Crow

Peter Mitchell

The early morning sun scorches the air, stilling the moment as if suspending time. Crow lands on a dead tree branch and settles its wings. Stan sees his friend and smiles. He shifts his gaze back to the grove of olive trees in the side yard. The remaining fruit are small brown nuts. *Half the orchard still needs harvesting, and the olives have to be washed and soaked.* He regards his limbs. Raised veins like taut string run along his lean arms while his legs are epidemic-thin. *How will it get done?*

A peripheral movement attracts his attention. Crow moves to another tree. *Ach, ach, ach!* Its harsh call scatters phrases across the air.

'Yes, I know,' replies Stan. He sits down, the verandah meeting his bony arse in slow motion. Standing for more than five minutes these days tires his legs.

In the kitchen his partner Pat stands at the bench, his arms seesawing slowly as he cuts sandwiches for his lunch. His briefcase leans against the table.

The jagged edges of the bare grey boards poke into Stan. He repositions himself, becoming comfortable again. He hears several footfalls and turns his head.

'I'm going now,' says Pat, standing behind him.

Stan looks up into Pat's eyes. Concern velvets them.

'Okay, my love,' Stan says. 'Will you ring Al today about ploughing the southern paddock?'

'Uh-huh.'

'I'm wondering if fifty hectares of wheat will do,' says Stan. He remembers sitting in the air-conditioned cabin years earlier, the tractor making symmetrical rows, the discs like curling irons turning red soil.

'I'll ring him later today,' says Pat.

'Okay. Drive safely.'

'I will,' says Pat, ruffling Stan's thinning hair. 'Do you need anything from the chemist?'

'Not today.'

Pat pecks Stan on his lips. Now that Pat's in his early seventies, his knees click each time he bends down. He turns, picks up his briefcase and walks to the Falcon on the other side of the house. Stan looks into the distance.

~

Sydney, 1985. Rainbow lights arced through the night sky above Moore Park. The humidity was like molasses, sticky and sweet. The crowd clapped and cheered as the Mardi Gras floats passed by. Sweat glistened on Stan's chest, his arm around his date, Jock.

Their eyes had played cat-and-mouse games: staring at each other for ten long seconds, looking away then looking back, shining with lust. After fifteen minutes, Jock had approached Stan, his thick Scottish brogue noticeable immediately. 'Aye,' he'd said in answer to a question, his blue eyes jewelling, 'I'm here on holidays.'

They walked arm in arm towards Sydney Showground, their minds a fusion of technicolour. The high heels of a drag queen in front of them looked like the Red Queen's throne from *Alice in Wonderland.* Near the entrance to the showground, each of them took out a ticket from their back pockets and joined the queues.

While waiting, Stan thought about Pat in their house at Randwick. Pat's date for the night had arrived in the late afternoon.

Stan's thoughts shifted backwards. After eight years together, Pat had suggested a change: an open relationship. Stan's stomach had roiled with anxiety in response. Many hours of back-and-forth words had coloured the air in their bedroom and kitchen. Honesty was the key, Pat had insisted. Finally, Stan had agreed.

Yet small knots of concern still tightened his stomach. As he inched towards the showground entrance, his reflection morphed into the mosaic of his and Pat's past, present and future. He pictured the two of them in bed together the following weekend as they recounted their respective adventures.

Stan and Jock idled through the turnstiles, knots of men and women islanding the grounds. Conversations rustled the air. It was Jock's first time at the party; Stan's second. When they entered Dome, strobe lights rainbowed across the walls and over the ceiling, free-floating above the cavorting crowds.

~

Stan's reverie ends as he crawls to a nearby chair. Using it as a support, he lifts himself up slowly, his long legs unfolding with difficulty. For twenty seconds, he tests his balance. *They're okay.* He shuffles into the dining room and sits at the table. Bottles of Truvada and Kaletra lie at oblique angles in a glass bowl in its centre. Over the past five years, his days have been defined by antiretrovirals taken in the morning and afternoon, being driven to Sydney for consultations with his specialists, and allaying Pat's fears about his health.

His eyes revolve around the room. *All these years with Pat.* Vases dot shelves; photographs of family members adorn walls; jars of fruit preserves fill the pantry. *I should've written all this down.* He glances at an exercise book where he's written random memories. Now he can't hold a pen for more than a few minutes at a time.

His wallet lies on the table close to him. He opens it. Pat's photograph smiles up at him. He slides it out and places it to the right. Five years ago he had it reprinted, the newness of it still shining. When his health started deteriorating, he decided the photograph of his life partner needed reprinting, needed a glossy finish.

Jock's photograph also stares at Stan from the wallet. He takes it out and holds it in his hands. At the sides, it is worn from age.

~

For long hours they danced in Dome, sweat and exuberance enveloping them. Jock suggested taking a break. Stan's skin cooled with the fresh air. Standing with water bottles in their hands, the two men enjoyed the effervescent crowd.

'Your chest hair's got silver tinsel in it,' said Stan. He ran his fingers over Jock's chest, his strawberry-blond hair moth-like to touch. Stan licked his fingers, the salt of Jock's perspiration enticing his palette. 'So that's what you taste like,' he said as Jock playfully pushed him away.

Later that night, each of them wrote calligraphies of pleasure and affection to the other.

~

Stan looks around the kitchen and dining room. They constrict him as if their shapes form an arrow, leading to a diminishing point.

Turning around, he looks out the back door, the line of earth and sky several hundred metres away. *I'd rather be outside ploughing the southern paddock.*

~

Pat turns right onto the Wellington to Dubbo Road. Five mornings a week he drives along it, the time to plan the day ahead. *Remember to ring Al.* He slows down as he drives around a left-hand curve. *Ah, yeah. The appointment with the Department of Primary Industries rep.*

Recollections of Diagnosis Day, as he calls it, run through his memory like film in reverse. It was a Sunday afternoon. Winter 1985. Clouds like brushstrokes streaked across a faded blue sky. He and Stan were lying in a bath of warm water. Pat leaned against the end of it and massaged his partner's shoulders as Stan spoke about his visit to Sydney.

'And there's another thing,' Stan said.

'Hmm.' Pat had his eyes closed. His imagination levitated above the bubble of warmth.

For several minutes, there was a long, drawn-out silence between them.

Pat turns the steering wheel right, driving around a bend. On the side of the road, two crows peck at the carcass of a dead wallaby. It's a few metres from the gate of Emoh Ruo, a wheat-and-sheep property run by close friends of theirs. *That's one thing I like about crows—they clean up carrion.*

Straightening the wheel, Pat recollects the lengthening silence that hovered over the bath like an unknown threat. He shivers as he remembers Stan looking up at him, his eyes appealing as if for forgiveness.

'I went to my doctor in Sydney,' Stan said.

'Hmm.'

'Well, he did a blood test the previous time I saw him.'

Pat remembers the pebble above the bath, held by an invisible hand.

'Well, it came back HIV-positive.'

The pebble dropped, hitting the still pond of their lives like a boulder. Waves crashed over Pat. After twenty seconds, he resurfaced as questions crammed his imagination.

'Who do you think it was?' he asked.

'My Scottish mate.'

'Do you think I am?

Stan shook his head. 'I don't think so.'

'What's the prognosis?'

Stan remained silent, letting his love's question fade away.

Pat negotiates the last bend before the bridge over the Lachlan River. On the left, the caravan park is an oasis of green, striking a contrast to the surrounding hectares, the colour of bleached bones.

He turns the front-door key, the words *Rural Insurance* in black lettering on the clear glass. He switches on the computer, starts a shopping list and rings Al, their hired help.

~

'Crows,' says Stan to the air in front of him. They were a constant presence throughout his childhood and are now here in the closing days of his life.

Many years earlier, he read a book of Indigenous stories. In one from the Kulin nation in central Victoria, Crow is a trickster character. The story has stayed with him. Makes him take particular notice of crows on the farm and keep mental notes about them.

Stan imagines the virus as a trickster, an artful dodger, swindling his body and misleading the medical establishment. One day it was his friend, the next his foe, the third a variation on the two.

Killing a crow, even accidentally, is an ill omen. That philosophy is from his father, and it threaded through their lives on the family farm in central Queensland.

Stan walks slowly to the side verandah. During midmorning, it is a cool refuge with a lounge and square pillows, the colours of the rainbow. Pat and their neighbours from Emoh Ruo arranged it for him.

~

Pat is sitting at his desk. He left a message on Al's phone to call him back. Behind him, the computer hums, its resonance a comforting vibration. He stares out at the street, his head resting in the envelope of his palms.

A tear rolls down the dry skin of his face. *What if.* The two words sit in his mind. *What if I hadn't suggested an open relationship?* It's a question he's asked himself many times.

A knock at the office door ends his reflections. He looks up and sees a shadow at the door. *Ah, yes. The bloke from Primary Industries.* He stands and unlocks the door he deliberately left locked.

~

'Are you following me, Crow?' asks Stan as if addressing an imaginary audience.

Crow turns his head sideways, his white eyes gazing at Stan with curiosity.

Stan sinks into the soft upholstery of the lounge then arranges himself in as comfortable a position as possible. 'Are you calling me to follow you?'

His question floats across the hectares.

'Well,' he says, turning his head, 'maybe one day.' He extends his legs, the muscles stretching.

He pictures himself accompanying Crow. He sees Pat below on the back verandah, waving farewell as the two of them cavort in currents of air, flying towards the line of earth and sky.

'It won't be too long now,' says Stan. He rests his head on a pillow, closes his eyes and imagines the silken air of flight caressing his skin.

~

The lion in the sky sinks behind the line of buildings, the shadows lengthening. Pat locks the front door, feeling he's had a productive day. Al will come in two days' time to help with the ploughing.

As Pat drives back over the Lachlan River bridge, its wooden surface rumbles under the tyres. He turns the steering wheel left, negotiating the curve after the bridge. He floors the accelerator, a plan in mind, eagerness urging him home.

~

The kelpie's bark signals Pat's arrival. Stan opens his eyes and lifts his head from the pillows.

'Hallo, hallo,' shouts Pat. He rests his briefcase on the dining table and walks to the side verandah. 'Ah, there you are.' He bends slowly to kiss Stan on the lips. 'Have you had a shower today?'

Stan shakes his head several times.

'Okay,' says Pat, his idea unfolding.

In the bathroom, he places the plastic chair in the middle of the shower recess and turns the water on. He adjusts the hot and cold, testing the falling water with his finger. *Good. Not too hot for Stan's skin.* He walks back to the side verandah.

'What are you doing?' asks Stan as Pat helps him to his feet.

'I have a plan.'

The two of them shuffle through the house to the bathroom.

'Hold the railing,' orders Pat. He undresses Stan, places his clothes over the bath's side and turns him around. 'Now, move back slowly and sit in the chair.'

'What's your plan?' says Stan, looking up.

'We're going to shower together like we used to,' says Pat. He kisses Stan fully on his mouth. He throws his work clothes over a nearby chair. 'Before everything changed.'

Stan gazes at the tiled floor. He remembers their times before Crow flew close to their world: warm baths together on Sunday afternoons, post-Mardi Gras recollections at their house in Randwick. He looks up again at Pat, his brown eyes warm. 'Before our viral friend welcomed the crow into our lives,' he says.

Year Sixty-Eight

Callum Methven

My great-grandmother gave him ten bob a week, on one condition: he wouldn't take up smoking. He's turning eighty-three in January.

~

I get there just after five, tell him I can only stay for tea, that I have to go to uni to see my supervisor the next day. The sun hangs over the water, moves further south along the horizon every week I visit, and it's been another week.

Warneet is a muddy inlet on the northern shores of Western Port Bay: boats, seagulls, fishing off the pier. Dad once told me the mangrove swamps are the southernmost in the world, and I've never bothered to look it up.

The gates are open, and the noisy miners are chasing a magpie around the yard. I find Pa in the kitchen cutting capsicum into the slow cooker, red in the face and his glasses fogged grey. I give him a hug and ask how he's been.

'All right, all right,' he says.

'How's Norm?'

'Clocked out Sunday night.'

'Bugger.'

'Yeah, smoked since he was fifteen, though. Good innings. He went fast, clinging on with enough morphine to take down a stud.'

I ask him how he is again, as if he didn't hear me the first time, and he says he's fine. It might even be true.

~

I told my housemate I'd go and get a haircut first, tackle my last assignment with a fresh head. My aunt is my hairdresser, up the road from the hospital where Nan was. Half of the oldies on the swamp end up in that hospital.

Afterwards my aunt and I decided to nick down and see Nan, just a quick visit, then I'd get home and finish my work. My aunt went to grab us coffees, so I was the first one there.

The hospital is a one-storey complex ringed around a garden where the patients get to walk when the weather is right. The weather was right that last Tuesday in October, but the only people I saw walking around were wearing pale-green scrubs. I could tell they loved their jobs.

When I got to Nan's room, Pa was waiting for me, Nan fast asleep. By his side was the palliative care nurse. It was the first time I'd ever seen my grandfather cry. He knew exactly what was going to happen.

Soon afterwards my aunt came in with the coffees. I don't really remember what happened after that.

~

'I want to go home.' Nan had this defiant look on her face every time she said it.

That's not where it started—and not where it ended, either—but for a long time all Nan wanted was to go home.

At first there were just small signs: a puzzled sigh, a vacant gaze. It was as if every room she walked into wasn't real, just déjà vu, but she never let on. Pa was the first one to notice it. I guess it made sense—she'd been by his side since he was fifteen. He knew what was happening; sixty-seven years is a very long time.

Home changed from here to there. Sometimes it was the old farm down in Koo Wee Rup, a hundred acres on the tip of Western Port Bay where she'd raised three kids, and sometimes it was the house of her own childhood down the valley.

We would take her for a drive to get some ice cream by the bridge in the nearby town of Tooradin, then drive her back home while she licked her lips. 'Yes, Nan,' we'd say, 'this is your house. It's a nice house, isn't it?' That seemed to help.

Last summer I was sitting with Nan and Pa outside their caravan, parked in my parents' back yard between the house and the pool—an annual tradition. The surrounding paddocks had faded yellow in the heat, and every now and again a cloud passed over, threatening rain. Nan watched the birds with a cuppa in her hands and waved at whoever happened to be in the kitchen window.

Pa had his own cuppa, and a big goofy smile was smeared across his face. 'I tucked her into bed yesterday,' he told me, 'and she said that she wanted to go home, so I asked her where home was. She said, 'Where the family is.' He turned to Nan. 'This is your family, isn't it?'

She smiled, nodded. 'Course it is,' she said, as if that was obvious.

~

When it wasn't sad, it was heartbreakingly funny.

Over a year went by before she passed. I used to sit by the window at their house and read while the tide came in or out. One day Nan edged over, hands behind her back, to stand in front of the fire. She waited until she had my eye. 'So,' she said, 'what was your last name again?'

I was caught off guard, but it was all I could do not to laugh. Her expression was confident, and I could tell she knew that she'd forgotten; she was trying to plod along and bluff. I put my book down, looked up with a smile. 'Well, Nan, guess what?'

'What?'

'My last name … is the same as yours.'

'Really?'

'Yep. Know why? It's because your son … is my dad. That's why I call you "Nan".'

Cheekiness bloomed across her face. 'Well,' she said, 'isn't that just good.'

By the time her eightieth birthday came around the following May, things were worse, but she was still herself. She didn't believe for a moment that she was eighty, but that just meant she was delighted to be receiving the same presents as she ate her meal.

He had bags under his eyes all the time.

~

Nan went to bed at nine every night, even if she wasn't to go to sleep for another six hours. She could see spiders on the walls, people at the door, even with the lights out. Pa would get the bug spray, tell her no one was there but her boy upstairs. She held his hand tight.

I saw Pa at six every morning when I came downstairs. It was usually still dark, first light coming after the blue light from the kettle. Sometimes the tide was up to the kangaroo grass, sometimes it was flat mud almost all the way to the mangroves on Quail Island.

'I've had me girl since I was fifteen and she was thirteen,' he'd say, 'that's sixty-seven years. No one gets sixty-seven years.'

He wasn't wrong, but it didn't seem to make anything better.

He was tired then, although some of that comes with age. He needed a break, the kind of real rest you have after never being able to shut your eyes. He couldn't let her out of his sight for weeks on end.

She was still Nan. Nan who'd had her first child at the age of nineteen. Nan who got up early to milk the cows for the forty years since she was old enough to go to school. Nan who walked into a bar to ask for a job when things were slow on the farm, having never mixed a drink in her life.

Nan wanted to go home, and she wasn't going to wait for anyone to take her.

The first few times it was okay. She'd walk the old path, and Pa would ring up their friends who lived down the road, get them to catch her from the other direction before she got too far. But it wasn't always that easy a task. She'd only ever drag her feet in her slippers.

I was in the yard with Pa and Dad, stacking piles of wood from the rusting trailer. Mum was around the back doing the washing. I don't know how long it was before we realised Nan had disappeared, but I remember the feeling, the hollowness. Pa rang their friends, but she hadn't gone past yet. Dad and I did a lap of town in the car.

We found her facedown in the lane where she used to walk us

to the general store—me, my siblings and my cousins—and we'd lick the melted ice cream from our sticky hands and race each other home.

Nan was bleeding on her hands, and her nose was swollen, but we didn't have to call the ambulance. A few weeks later she was admitted to the hospital after falling out of bed in the middle of the night; a few weeks after that came the nursing home.

~

The clock on the wall showed it was two in the morning. The never-ending plethora of b-list nineties horror movies on the TV reminded us it was Halloween. I sat with my cousin making banal jokes about the bizarre world of early morning television, and Pa sat next to us in Nan's chair, his sleeping wife gripping his hand whenever the nurses turned her over to face him. The tears had turned to laughter, which had turned to a peculiar version of purgatory in which time was an idea and the only constant was an occasional visit from one of the staff.

Nan didn't stir, and Pa didn't sleep. 'I'm just glad we got her in the right place,' he kept saying.

He wasn't wrong: the staff were pretty amazing. Considering that death is a part of the job, they were an awfully cheerful bunch. They let themselves care about people who they knew would likely die soon, and when it happened they would be right back in the next shift ready for a new patient.

At the start of that Tuesday, none of us had known it was going to be the longest day of our lives. It lasted all the way through to Saturday.

I woke up the morning after it was over to my brother knocking on my bedroom window from outside, grey marks beneath his eyes. On the way back to our parents' we listened to a song called 'It's Nice to Be Alive'.

~

It's the day after Christmas, and the sun is burning through a giant hole in the ozone layer. I come inside from the dry December heat and sit myself down next to Pa on the couch. The rumpus room still smells like a dying pine. On the TV two men in white pants run up and down a strip of bald grass; it's the Boxing Day Test.

I fluff Pa's grey hair around and fashion it into a mohawk. He elbows me in the ribs and tells me the score to a day I haven't been following. I say something about a good Christmas, and he agrees. He's nearly two months into whatever happens after the rest of your life, and at this point I'm wondering what comes next.

Eventually both teams break, and the game is stopped where it is. Sometimes we talk about it, but today I just ask Pa why they've stopped playing.

'Must be done for the day, I guess,' he says, 'but they'll be back tomorrow.'

He's not wrong. And they'll be back there next year too.

Snowdrops

Rachel Burns

In the garden she noticed the stooped white heads of snowdrops. The crocuses were starting to come up through the loose soil, they poked their purple buds, tested the air. There was something wonderful about early spring flowers, year upon year; it always surprised her.

Earlier she heard a woman scream, somewhere on the housing estate. The sound found her on her walk, a real visceral cry of despair, and it haunted her. She'd once screamed like that, when she'd found him in a crumpled heap, collapsed at the bottom of the stairs, the telephone table knocked sideways.

It could be something or nothing—hysteria, she reasoned with herself. Some women, she thought, are hysterical all the time for no good reason. Her grandmother had been a formidable woman who had terrible rages over spilt milk or burnt toast, or even an article in the newspaper. Her grandfather used to try and make light of it. 'Hormones,' he would say, as he ducked a flying plate.

Strange then, irrational even, that she kept her ears pricked for the sound of a siren as she walked with a purposeful stride across the farmer's muddy field. Her wellington boots squelched in a satisfying way. She was careful to hold her breath as she went past the sewage yard, the pungency of raw effluent so powerful it made her nauseous. The physical act of holding her breath brought back memories of Jack Senior: his constant wheezing, the strange sound he'd made like a worn-out hymn.

The path was difficult to negotiate because of all the rain, which had been relentless for months, and she was tired of mud splattering her clothes and of not being able to walk at a faster pace. She thought back to the scream; it reminded her of a line from a Sylvia Plath poem, something about a woman in an ambulance and a red heart. But there were no sirens, there was no ambulance that rushed to an emergency, and she reprimanded herself in the loud stern voice her mother would have used, 'Really, Susan, you *are* silly, what fanciful ideas you have.'

Her dog was running wild in the woods somewhere; she heard the odd startled rasping sound of a pheasant flushed from its hiding place, followed by an eerie silence. The dog seemed to disappear completely. She listened to the elms, their branches creaking in the wind, diseased trunks that knocked against each other. Her stomach knotted; she was a woman wholly alone in the woods.

When the two of them appeared, she was startled, her heart bounced in her chest. A man in a red beanie hat was walking with a young boy, who she guessed was about eight, a slight, skinny child. Then her dog reappeared, running about them like a jack-in-the-box, weaving in and out of their legs like a thing possessed. She crossly called the dog to heel and shouted an apology to the man and his boy. She presumed it was his boy; she wondered what they were doing in the woods. Shouldn't the boy be in school? Perhaps he was sick. He didn't look sick—pasty, yes, but not sick enough to warrant a day off.

The dog was deliberately ignoring her commands, and ran between the boy's legs, then jumped up at the man as if expecting a treat. At last, she was able to snatch the dog by the collar, and the man said to the boy as they both passed, 'Boy, he's excitable.'

The boy, laughing, said, 'Yes.'

She relaxed then—obviously just a father and his son taking a stroll through the woods.

She remembered being with her grandfather when she was a girl, and the bluebells. Gosh, yes, the bluebells, armfuls to take back to her grandmother, and the smell of wild garlic as she knelt to pick the flowers.

Her grandfather worshipped the outdoors. 'Anyone would,' he often said, 'after years spent on hands and knees, crawling along coal seams in the dark.' He had been a miner after leaving school at fifteen, then suddenly the mines were all gone.

They would play Pooh sticks in the beck, stopping at the little bridges that crossed the railway line. He would tell her about the steam trains, about how when he was a boy, his mother used to send him down to collect the black lumps that fell off the backs of coal wagons.

She had visions of her grandfather as a small boy on the tracks as a steam train hurtled towards him. 'Wasn't that dangerous?' she'd ask.

His eyes gleamed, and he replied, 'Very dangerous, yes.'

He made bows and arrows out of branches and sharpened the ends with a knife. She remembered he always had a piece of wood in his hands; he was forever whittling something, strangely shaped little animals and mythical creatures.

Another trick he showed from time to time was to pick a handful of nettles and crunch them in his bare hands. He was immune to stings and recounted a story about how his father had kept beehives: one day, when he was only small, he was attacked by the whole hive and very nearly died.

Sometimes she forgot her grandfather was no longer alive.

There was something about the man and the boy, the way they carried themselves, the long sticks they used as walking poles. The man looked like he was making a real effort, perhaps showing the boy his childhood, perhaps saying, *These are the woods I played in as a boy.*

She was back to the sewage yard, the work van was parked up, and she thought perhaps this area was not as isolated as one might think—deceptively so, even. Plenty of people came and went, plenty of people on mobile phones. Then, once again, she was crossing the backs of houses where she'd heard the terrible scream. There was no sound of anything untoward. *Hysteria, then*, she thought. *Nothing more.*

~

In the quiet of the afternoon, she is listened to a news programme on the local radio station and argued with the guest speaker even though they couldn't hear her. 'What a ridiculous thing to say. How would you know? You're not even married.'

Next, she aired out the bedrooms, straightened the beds, even the ones that hadn't been slept in for years, opened the windows, let in the fresh air. She spotted black mildew growing around the window in Jack Junior's room and made a mental note to bleach it later, she knew she would put it off for weeks because she hated the powerful smell of ammonia. It reminded her too much of hospitals.

Then she did the day's washing-up; she liked to leave her breakfast and dinner plates in the sink to soak and do the whole lot after supper. She had allowed herself to do this for some time, grown accustomed to the mess malaudering in the sink. She picked 'malaudering' up from her mother; she didn't even think it was a real word.

When the washing-up was done, dried and put away, she sat in the kitchen chair and watched the sky gradually darken. The radio presenter talked about the day's events, the same old headlines of police corruption and budget cuts. She found she was listening more intently than usual.

She didn't know why she thought there might be a terrible announcement: a missing boy, a stabbing, a bloodstained knife. Then her mind wandered off, and she imagined she was walking through the woods again, this time accompanied by a nice young policeman about her son's age. She was showing him exactly where she saw the young boy strolling with that man. Oh yes, she could describe him very accurately: mid-twenties, a red beanie hat, medium build, brown hair, brown eyes. 'That is what struck me,' she said, 'the eyes. They were frantic eyes, those of someone running scared.'

~

She'd been lost in thought for some time when her mobile phone rang—the Shostakovich tune, the one that everyone knew. Jack Junior downloaded it for her when he purchased the phone. She hadn't the heart to tell him how much she hated Shostakovich; it was music that belonged to Jack Senior, not her.

'Hello, Mum.'

'Oh, Jack Junior, it's you.' Her son always rang on Tuesday evenings at seven o'clock. He worried if she didn't answer. She looked out of the window, surprised to see that it was dark already.

'Please don't call me that, Mum. You okay?'

'Oh dear,' she glanced at the kitchen clock, 'is that the time already?' She suddenly felt very tired.

'Sorry, Mum, is it a bad time? Do you want me to ring back later?'

'No, no, it's lovely to hear your voice, you know what I'm like. I was away with the fairies.'

They laughed together, a little conspiratorial laugh.

When Jack Senior was alive, he used to get so cross. She remembered that he used to think they were laughing at him. It was as if he was jealous that she and Jack Junior had something between them he couldn't quite grasp.

She told Jack Junior about her day, about the blood-curdling scream and the strange man (for now in her imagination he had grown strange) with the little boy who should have been in school.

'It's probably nothing, Mum.'

His voice reassured her; he was right, of course. She spent far too much time on her own, letting her imagination run away with her.

~

She opened the patio doors and let the dog out into the garden; it was a clear night, and she could see the stars, the waxing gibbous moon. She remembered nights like this when Jack Senior was in the hospital, those clear nights when she gazed out of the window from Ward 23, and marvelled at the night sky, listened to her husband struggle to breathe, the sound of the oxygen machine and the magnified ticking of the clock.

She remembered the harassed social worker who talked to her at the hospital. 'Being a full-time carer isn't easy.'

If only she knew. Jack Senior's temper had got worse as his shortness of breath slowly deteriorated, eventually reaching the point where he couldn't even manage the stairs. But he was adamant he was not going to sleep on the sofa bed downstairs.

She watched him, stubborn as a mule, climbing to the top, clean out of breath, his face turning blue. 'Help me, Woman.' He could barely get the words out; she could barely hear him.

She should have gone to help him, at least fetched the nebuliser, but she just stood there and watched. She was worn out with it all, the constant call to duty. She was looking forward to taking the dog for a walk in the fresh air. Thirty minutes of peace, away from him.

It was a shock when he fell, his body crashed down the stairs, his head hit the telephone table, knocking it sideways, his crumpled heap, the stunned silence.

Then there was the scream, that terrible scream, that came from deep inside her.

At first she was terrified he was dead, but then something kicked in, and she was checking his pulse, faint but still there. In slow motion she picked up the telephone stand then the telephone, placed it back on the table and dialled 999.

'Ambulance, please.' Her voice was detached, as calm as anything.

There was a great deal of blood where he had bashed his head. Her heart thumped so she could feel it in her rib cage, yet she managed to find a clean tea towel. She sat and cradled his head as they waited for the ambulance to arrive, the blood seeped into the white cloth like a rose in bloom. He lost consciousness and came around only fleetingly; she'd never forgotten the look in his eyes.

A few days in the hospital, a machine to help him breathe, then the decision not to revive. Jack Junior said it was the right thing to do.

She let the dog back into the house from the garden, locked the doors and made her way upstairs to bed. She closed the sash-window, cleaned her teeth at the little sink, undressed, put on her nightie and climbed into her side of the bed. She loved this time of the evening, the smell and feel of cool aired sheets against her skin. With the clear night sky imprinted on her brain, she drifted off into a deep sleep.

Contributors

Reinfred Dziedzorm Addo is a Ghanaian-American writer/speech-language pathologist currently residing in Gainesville, Florida. Reinfred's medical creative writing has been published by the US National Foundation of Swallowing Disorders. His general creative writing has appeared in *Land and territory: An anthology, Tampered Press* and *Masques*. Reinfred is working towards publishing his first-ever poetry collection.

Leah Baker resides in Portland, Oregon, and teaches writing at a public high school. Her writing has been featured or is forthcoming in *Pointed Circle, For Women Who Roar, Voice Catcher* and *Thirty West Publishing*. She is a current PhD student at the California Institute for Integral Studies.

Emily Bourne is an artist, freelance writer and activist from London. She enjoys making art surrounding LGBTIQ+ issues and disability rights. She's currently an editor at a small online e-magazine called *Risen Zine* and hopes to work in the journalism sector in the future. Keep up with what she's doing by following her Instagram: @floteren.

Rachel Burns is from Durham City, England. Her short stories are published in *Mslexia* and *Here Comes Everyone*. Her poetry pamphlet *A Girl in a Blue Dress* is available from Vane Women Press. You can follow her on Twitter: @RachelLBurnsme.

Josie Byrne is a playwright from Bolton, England. She is the artistic director of the On the Go Theatre Group. Her plays include *Cotton Queen*, *Someone's Sons*, *Word of War* and *Dirty Face*. Her latest play *You Have Never Had It So Good* about life in the 1950s is waiting to be rehearsed and performed after the global pandemic ends.

Ann Calandro was born and raised in New York, NY. She is a retired medical editor, a mixed media collage artist, a writer, and a classical piano student. Her writings have been published in *The Fabulist, Lou Lit, Duck Lake Journal, University of Windsor Review* and other journals, and her artwork has been exhibited in galleries and included in *Mud Season Review*, *The Penn Review*, *Memoir Magazine* and *NUNUM*, among other publications. She lives in New Jersey.

Al Campbell is a Brisbane-based part-time academic researcher and editor, and a full-time parent/carer of two young men on the autistic spectrum. Also: a 4 a.m. writer. Al used to act a bit, long ago. Her short fiction has been published in *Overland*. 'Does he feel warm?' is an extract from her debut novel, *The Things of This World*, to be released by UQP in 2022. You can follow her on Twitter: @aa_campbell.

Steve Cushman's story 'Fracture City' first appeared in the collection *Fracture City* (Main Street Rag Publishing, 2008). Steve has also published three novels. His first full-length poetry collection, *'How Birds Fly'*, is the winner of the 2018 Lena Shull Book Award. After twenty years as an X-ray technologist, Steve now works in healthcare IT.

Scott Dalgarno counts himself fortunate to have seen his essays and poems appear in *American Poetry Review*, *Yale Review, Antioch Review, Bellevue Literary Review, Pilgrimage, The Christian Century*, *Presbyterians Today and Presbyterian Outlook*. He served six churches over thirty years in Oregon and is now in his tenth year as pastor of Wasatch Presbyterian Church in Salt Lake City, Utah.

Katie Danis studies medical anthropology at the University of North Carolina at Chapel Hill. Her poem 'Dissecting Your Dad' won the Walker Percy Prize for excellence in medical humanities writing and was published in the Health Humanities Journal of UNC Chapel Hill (Spring 2020 edition).

D.E.L. writes personal essays and intends to publish a collection of experiences on mental health and supernatural phenomena. D.E.L. thrives as bipolar and as a single mama. She thanks her family, dog and therapist, and the many beautiful people she has met on her journey, especially her daughter, Ava Ming, who makes her world go 'round. You can follow her on Instagram: @dana_eileenthe_queen.

Jann Everard's short fiction has been published in Canada, the United States, and New Zealand. Recent and forthcoming work can be found in *The New Quarterly*, *Humber Literary Review*, *Belmont Story Review*, *Prairie Fire* and *EVENT*. Jann was the winner of *The Malahat Review's* 2018 Open Season Award for Fiction. She lives in Toronto, Canada.

Darci Flatley earned her MFA in Writing from the University of San Francisco and now works in the non-profit sector to house homeless youth. She was raised outside of Jacksonville, Florida, and spent her childhood exploring and roughhousing with her two siblings. When not writing, Darci enjoys reading, gardening, and a good cup of tea. This is her first publication.

Annette Freeman is a writer living in Sydney, Australia. She has a Master of Creative Writing degree, and her short fiction has been published in a number of international and Australian literary journals. She is working on a novel set in the backblocks of Tasmania. Annette tweets at @sendchampagne.

Rebecca Garnett Haris lives in London, UK, works in the NHS and is the mother of an autistic child. She is finishing her MA in Creative Writing at Teesside University and is currently working on an historical novel based on an autistic child in 1950s USA who is sent to an asylum.

Rukayatu Ibrahim is a pediatrician in the USA. She lives and works in the American Midwest. Originally from Ghana, West Africa, she went to medical school there and is hoping to build a pediatric practice in her home country in a hybrid virtual and in-person model at some point in the future. In her spare time, she writes fiction and listens to audiobooks (mostly realistic fiction but also non-fiction that interests her), watches travel documentaries and indie/quirky movies.

C.A. Limina is an Indonesian writer and undergraduate student. Their works have been featured in various media, including the *Jakarta Post* and *Kill Your Darlings*. Cal is pursuing a bachelor's degree in Petra Christian University's English department.

Vanessa Maclellan's first novel, *Three Great Lies*, was published by Hadley Rille Books in 2015. She's had seven works of fiction published, including a story in the *Young Explorer's Adventure Guide*. A member of SFWA and Codex, and a graduate of the Viable Paradise workshop, she writes, hikes, camps and bird watches in the Pacific Northwest, USA.

Callum Methven is a writer and translator from Bunyip, Australia. His poetry and short fiction have appeared in Monash University Publishing's *Verge* anthology, and he has a healthy predilection for science fiction. He is currently working on completing several novels in verse, as well as a poetry translation from Spanish.

Peter Mitchell is the author of *Conspiracy of Skin* (Ginninderra Press, 2018) and *The Scarlet Moment* (Picaro Press, 2009). Living in Lismore in Bundjalung Country, New South Wales, he writes short fiction, poetry, memoir and literary criticism. His memoir *Fragments through the Epidemic* awaits a publisher, and he is currently completing his first full poetry collection, *The Loam of Memory*.

Isabella Mori, who lives in Canada, is a counsellor and the author of two books of and about poetry, including *A bagful of haiku—87 imperfections*. Isabella's poetry, short stories and nonfiction have been published in places such as the anthology *The Group of Seven Reimagined*. She founded and organizes Muriel's Journey Poetry Prize, which celebrates loud, edgy, socially engaged poetry.

Sophie Overett is an award-winning writer, podcaster and cultural producer based in Melbourne, Australia. Her stories have been published around the world, and her podcast, *Lady Parts*, explores women in genre cinema. Her debut novel, *The Rabbits*, will be published by Penguin Australia in 2021.

C.A. Rivera is an American physician-writer from Los Angeles. His poetry has appeared or is forthcoming in the *Garfield Lake Review*, *Ars Medica*, *Body Electric*, and elsewhere. He was a participant at the Bread Loaf Writers Conference. He lives in Los Angeles with his family, where he is a practicing gastroenterologist and working on a collection of short stories.

Janey Runci is a fiction writer at Meat Market Studio Program in Melbourne. Her short stories have been published in literary journals, magazines and anthologies including *Best Australian Stories*. She has won prizes for her fiction in a number of Australian competitions, and in the international Bridport and Fish competitions. She is working on a collection of linked stories.

Sarah Sasson is a physician-writer from Sydney, Australia. Her poetry, short stories and creative non-fiction have been published in Australia, the UK and USA, appearing in *Meanjin, Oxford Writers' House*, *Medium*, *Unsweetened*, *Grieve Anthology*, *Intersection Stories*, *Translating Pain* and *Orris Root*. Her work explores themes including human relationships, memory, medicine and biology.

Nicole Zelniker (she/her) is a writer, activist and podcast producer at The Nasiona. She is also the author of *Mixed*, a non-fiction book about race and mixed-race families, and *Last Dance*, a collection of short stories. Check out the rest of her work at nicolezelniker.com.

Editor's Acknowledgements

I would like to firstly acknowledge and pay my respects to the Bidgigal and Gadigal people of the Eora Nation, the Traditional Custodians of the land on which I live on, and on which this anthology was edited.

Thank you to Melanie van Kessel, whose art features on the *Signs of Life* website and cover: for beautiful work and inspiring collaboration.

Thank you to the nearly 200 writers who answered the call-out and submitted their pieces. It was a privilege to read your words and confirmed to me that the talent pool of emerging writers is both wide and deep. Whittling down the submissions to a stand-out longlist and eventual selection was made difficult by the high standard of your work.

To the 25 contributors: you are all writers of exceptional talent working on subjects that matter. Thank you for believing in this project; the stories you have shared mean a great deal to me and I will carry them forward, within me, for many years to come. You all displayed great courtesy and professionalism, even when the past year put additional strains on us all, and even when things like getting to a printer and having contracts witnessed were prevented by pandemic lockdowns. Thank you for making my journey as editor an enjoyable one. Special thanks to Jann Everard and Al Campbell for additional eleventh-hour assistance, in providing feedback on my piece.

To my copyeditor Kate Goldsworthy, with whom it is a pleasure and privilege to work with—thank you for again letting me hold the scalpel, but for always pointing tactfully and showing me where to cut.

Thank you to Michelle Johnston for a generosity of spirit and of words.

Thank you to Sophie McNamara: for friendship, encouragement and editorial advice.

Finally, I would like to express my sincere thanks and loving gratitude to my husband Chris Andersen, who has always provided unwavering support for all of my ventures, both within medicine, and beyond.

Index

Printed in Great Britain
by Amazon

60150847R00113